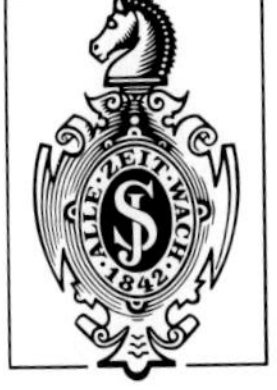
ALLE · ZEIT · WACH
1842

M. Kitahara (Ed.)

Ménière's Disease

With 101 Illustrations

Springer-Verlag
Tokyo Berlin Heidelberg
New York London Paris
Hong Kong Barcelona

Masaaki Kitahara, M.D.
Director, The Vestibular Disorder Research Committee
Professor and Head, Department of Otolaryngology, Shiga University of Medical Science,
Seta, Otsu, 520-21 Japan

ISBN 4-431-70056-0 Springer-Verlag Tokyo Berlin Heidelberg New York
ISBN 3-540-70056-0 Springer-Verlag Berlin Heidelberg New York Tokyo
ISBN 0-387-70056-0 Springer-Verlag New York Berlin Heidelberg Tokyo

Library of Congress Cataloging-in-Publication Data
Ménière's disease / M. Kitahara (ed.). p. cm. Includes bibliographical references. Includes index.
ISBN 4-431-70056-0 ISBN 3-540-70056-0 ISBN 0-387-70056-0 1. Ménière's disease.
I. Kitahara, Masaaki. [DNLM: 1. Meniere's Disease—diagnosis. 2. Meniere's Disease—physiopathology. 3. Meniere's Disease—therapy. WV 258 M5452] RF275.M44 1990 617.8′82—dc20
DNLM/DLC 90-10153

Typesetting: Asco Trade Typesetting Ltd., Hong Kong
Printing: Kowa Art Printing, Tokyo
Binding: Kubota Binding, Tokyo

Preface

Ménière's disease is often a wastebasket diagnosis for conditions of dizziness of unknown origin. To guide physicians in making a diagnosis, it would be desirable for this ailment to have a common base for management as many other specific diseases have. Ménière's is certainly a disease with unknown etiology, and it is quite difficult to determine its origin, a fact recognized by all investigators in the world, without exception. However, there is no excuse for the fact that this ailment is still a dumping ground for dizziness which cannot be neatly associated with something else. It is too easy to state that the complete story was given by Ménière himself, his description has never been improved upon, and everything is still speculative until we acquire more knowledge. For an intractable ailment such as Ménière's disease, however, it is probable that an endless chain of unknown etiologies will continue even though occasional origins are confirmed in some cases. Therefore, our knowledge must be constantly updated in order that physicians may obtain the greatest benefit from it. When the picture of Ménière's disease becomes clearer through this compilation, the investigations of the etiology of this ailment will continue in the right direction.

The Ministry of Health and Welfare of Japan designated as "intractable" 43 diseases of which the etiology is unknown and for which definitive treatment methods are not yet established. For each of these diseases, a research committee was organized and intensive investigations are being carried out with the aid of grants from the Ministry. The Vestibular Disorder Research Committee, formerly known as the Ménière's Disease Research Committee, has designed and proceeded with research on Ménière's disease, which was designated "intractable" in 1974. The present volume consists of recent studies resulting from the activities of our committee. It is my wish that this volume will help promote interest in the problems of Ménière's disease and encourage those physicians who have been confronted with this difficult ailment.

The encouragement and help I have received in the achievement of the study and publication of this volume comes from too many sources to mention here. However, I would especially like to express my heartfelt appreciation and gratitude to Professor Emeritus of Osaka University, Toshi Naito, M.D., Professor Emeritus of Tokyo Medical and Dental University, Isamu Watanabe, M.D., and Former Professor of Kyoto University, Manabi Hinoki, M.D., for their enthusiastic help and advice in our research of Ménière's disease. Dr. T. Naito is a disciple of Professor Emeritus of Osaka University, Kyoshiro Yamakawa, M.D., who first revealed the pathological findings of Ménière's disease in 1938, and of Professor George Portmann, M.D., who invented endolymphatic sac drainage surgery for Ménière's disease in 1927. Dr. J.J. Shea recognized Naito's leadership in *Laryngoscope* (89:1244–1256, 1979). Dr. T. Naito first created endolymphatic hydrops in guinea pigs by the obliteration of the endolymphatic sac and by other techniques in 1950. He also invented subarachnoid drainage surgery for Ménière's disease together with Dr. K. Yamakawa in 1952. Dr. T. Naito is indeed a pioneer of Ménière's disease study. Dr. I. Watanabe and Dr. M. Hinoki were directors of the Ménière's Disease Research Committee (1974–1979) and the Vestibular Disorder Research Committee (1980–1985), respectively. They have influenced the development of Ménière's disease research in Japan and made special efforts to establish its current stature. I am also deeply grateful to our committee members for their cooperation in our research project and to the Disease Control Division of the Health Service Bureau, the Ministry of Health and Welfare, Japan, for its enormous service in promoting our activities.

Masaaki Kitahara

Contents

Part IV. Treatment of Ménière's Disease

Part V. Other Diseases with Endolymphatic Hydrops

List of Contributors

K. Akioka, M.D.,
Department of Otolaryngology, Nara Medical College, Shijo-cho, Kashihara, 634 Japan

E. Arakawa, M.D.,
Department of Otolaryngology, Tohoku University School of Medicine, Seiryo-cho, Sendai, 980 Japan

S. Aso, M.D.,
Department of Otolaryngology, Faculty of Medicine, Toyama Medical and Pharmaceutical University, Sugitani, Toyama, 930-01 Japan

N. Fujita, M.D.,
Department of Otolaryngology, Nara Medical College, Shijo-cho, Kashihara, 634 Japan

F. Fujiwara, M.D.,
Department of Otolaryngology, Hirosaki University School of Medicine, Zaifu-cho, Hirosaki, 036 Japan

K. Fukuoka, M.D.,
Department of Otolaryngology, Hirosaki University School of Medicine, Zaifu-cho, Hirosaki, 036 Japan

E. Fukushi, M.D.,
Department of Otolaryngology, Hirosaki University School of Medicine, Zaifu-cho, Hirosaki, 036 Japan

Y. Furuhashi, M.D.,
Department of Otolaryngology, University of Tsukuba Institute of Clinical Medicine, Tennodai, Tsukuba, 305 Japan

M. Furuta, M.D.,
Department of Pathology, Kyoto Takeda Hospital, Shimogyo, Kyoto, 606 Japan

A. Hara, M.D.,
Department of Otolaryngology, Tsukuba University Institute of Clinical Medicine, Tennodai, Tsukuba, 305 Japan

J. Handa, M.D.,
Professor, Department of Neurosurgery, Shiga University of Medical Science, Seta, Otsu, 520-21 Japan

J. Hozawa, M.D.,
Professor, Department of Otolaryngology, Hirosaki University School of Medicine, Zaifu-cho, Hirosaki, 036 Japan

K. Hozawa, M.D.,
Department of Otolaryngology, Tohoku University School of Medicine, Seiryo-cho, Sendai, 980 Japan

M. Ikeda, M.D.,
Section of Otolaryngology, Soka City Hospital, Soka, 340 Japan

K. Ikeno, M.D.,
Department of Otolaryngology, Hirosaki University School of Medicine, Zaifu-cho, Hirosaki, 036 Japan

T. Inamori, M.D.,
Assistant Professor, Department of Otolaryngology, Hyogo College of Medicine, Mukogawa-cho, Nishinomiya, 663 Japan

T. Ishii, M.D.,
Professor, Department of Otolaryngology, Tokyo Women's Medical College, Kawada-cho, Shinjuku-ku, Tokyo, 162 Japan

Z. Ito, M.D.,
Department of Otolaryngology, University of Tsukuba Institute of Clinical Medicine, Tennodai, Tsukuba, 305 Japan

H. Iwasaki, M.D.,
2-41-105 Saidaijiminami-cho, Nara, 631 Japan

T. Kamimura, M.D.,
Department of Medicine, Hirosaki University School of Medicine, Zaifu-cho, Hirosaki, 036 Japan

T. Kawase, M.D.,
Department of Otolaryngology, Tohoku University School of Medicine, Seiryo-cho, Sendai, 980 Japan

S. Kishimoto, M.D.,
Associate Professor, Department of Otolaryngology, Kochi Medical School, Nangoku, 781-51 Japan

M. Kitahara, M.D.,
Professor, Department of Otolaryngology, Shiga University of Medical Science, Seta, Otsu, 520-21 Japan

H. Kitano, M.D.,
Department of Otolaryngology, Shiga University of Medical Science, Seta, Otsu, 520-21 Japan

Y. Kitaoku, M.D.,
Department of Otolaryngology, Nara Medical College, Shijo-cho, Kashihara, 634 Japan

H. Kobayashi, M.D.,
Assistant Professor, Department of Otolaryngology, Faculty of Medicine, Toyama Medical and Pharmaceutical University, Sugitani, Toyama, 930-01 Japan

T. Kobayashi, M.D.,
Department of Otolaryngology, Tohoku University School of Medicine, Seiryo-cho, Sendai, 980 Japan

I. Koh, M.D.,
Department of Otolaryngology, Nara Medical College, Shijo-cho, Kasihara, 634 Japan

T. Kumoi, M.D.,
Professor, Department of Otolaryngology, Hyogo College of Medicine, Mukogawa-cho, Nishinomiya, 663 Japan

J. Kusakari, M.D.,
Professor, Department of Otolaryngology, University of Tsukuba Institute of Clinical Medicine, Tennodai, Tsukuba, 305 Japan

T. Machida, Ph.D.,
Department of Mechanical Engineering, Tamagawa University, Tamagawa Gakuen, Machida, Tokyo, 194 Japan

H. Masutani, M.D.,
Department of Otolaryngology, Osaka City University Medical School, Asahi-cho, Abeno-ku, Osaka, 545 Japan

K. Matsunaga, M.D.,
Department of Otolaryngology, Osaka City University Medical School, Asahi-cho, Abeno-ku, Osaka, 545 Japan

T. Matsunaga, M.D.,
Professor, Department of Otolaryngology, Nara Medical College, Shijo-cho, Kashihara, 634 Japan

C. Mizukami, M.D.,
Department of Otolaryngology, Kobe City General Hospital, Minatojima-Nakamachi, Kobe, 650 Japan

K. Mizukoshi, M.D.,
Professor, Department of Otolaryngology, Faculty of Medicine, Toyama Medical and Pharmaceutical University, Sugitani, Toyama, 930-01 Japan

H. Mori, M.D.,
Assistant Professor, Department of Otolaryngology, Hyogo College of Medicine, Mukogawa-cho, Nishinomiya, 663 Japan

M. Moriguchi, M.D.,
Department of Otolaryngology, Osaka City University Medical School, Asahi-cho, Abeno-ku, Osaka, 545 Japan

Y. Nakai, M.D.,
Professor, Department of Otolaryngology, Osaka City University Medical School, Asahi-cho, Abeno-ku, Osaka, 545 Japan

Y. Niizeki, M.D.,
Section of Otolaryngology, Kudanzaka Hospital, Tokyo, 102 Japan

N. Nishikawa, M.D.,
Department of Otolaryngology, University of Tsukuba Institute of Clinical Medicine, Tennodai, Tsukuba, 305 Japan

K. Ohta, M.D.,
Department of Otolaryngology, Mimuro Prefectural Hospital, Mimuro Sango-cho, 634 Japan

K. Ohyama, M.D.,
Department of Otolaryngology, Tohoku University School of Medicine, Seiryo-cho, Sendai, 980 Japan

H. Otani, M.D.,
Department of Anatomy, Shimane Medical University, Izumo, 693 Japan

M. Rokugo, M.D.,
Department of Otolaryngology, Tohoku University School of Medicine, Seiryo-cho, Sendai, 980 Japan

H. Saito, M.D.,
Professor, Department of Otolaryngology, Kochi Medical School, Nangoku, 781-51 Japan

I. Sawada, M.D.,
Department of Otolaryngology, Shiga University of Medical Science, Seta, Otsu, 520-21 Japan

H. Shinohara, M.D.,
Department of Anatomy, Shimane Medical University, Izumo, 693 Japan

H. Shojaku, M.D.,
Department of Otolaryngology, Faculty of Medicine, Toyama Medical and Pharmaceutical University, Sugitani, Toyama, 930-01 Japan

M. Sugita, M.D.,
Department of Otolaryngology, Osaka City University Medical School, Asahi-cho, Abeno-ku, Osaka, 545 Japan

M. Suzuki, M.D.,
Department of Otolaryngology, Shiga University of Medical Science, Seta, Otsu, 520-21 Japan

T. Takeda, M.D.,
Associate Professor, Department of Otolaryngology, Kochi Medical School, Nangoku, 781-51 Japan

M. Takeyama, M.D.,
Department of Otolaryngology, Tsukuba University Institute of Clinical Medicine, Tennodai, Tsukuba, 305 Japan

H. Tanaka, M.D.,
Department of Otolaryngology, Shiga University of Medical Science, Seta, Otsu, 520-21 Japan

O. Tanaka, M.D.,
Professor, Department of Anatomy, Shimane Medical University, Izumo, 693 Japan (Chapter 13)

O. Tanaka, M.D.,
Department of Otolaryngology, Nara Medical College, Shijo-cho, Kashihara, 634 Japan (Chapter 9)

K. Uchida, M.D.,
Department of Otolaryngology, Shiga University of Medical Science, Seta, Otsu, 520-21 Japan

Y. Wada, M.D.,
Department of Otolaryngology, Nara Medical College, Shijo-cho, Kashihara, 634 Japan

I. Watanabe, M.D.,
Emeritus Professor, Neuro-Otological Research Laboratory, 3-17-14 Yushima, Bunkyo-ku, Tokyo, 113 Japan

Y. Watanabe, M.D.,
Associate Professor, Department of Otolaryngology, Faculty of Medicine, Toyama Medical and Pharmaceutical University, Sugitani, Toyama, 930-01 Japan

E. Yamamoto, M.D.,
Director, Department of Otolaryngology, Kobe City General Hospital, Minatojima-Nakamachi, Kobe, 650 Japan

N. Yamamoto, M.D.,
Department of Otolaryngology, Tokyo Women's Medical College, Kawada-cho, Shinjuku-ku, Tokyo, 162 Japan

Y. Yazawa, M.D.,
Assistant Professor, Department of Otolaryngology, Shiga University of Medical Science, Seta, Otsu, 520-21 Japan

Part I. Introduction

CHAPTER 1

Concepts and Diagnostic Criteria of Ménière's Disease

Masaaki Kitahara

In 1861, Prosper Ménière [1] reported the gross pathological findings in a young girl who died after suffering from vertigo, tinnitus, and deafness. He found bloody exudate in her semicircular canals. Though some carelessness was noted in his reports on this case, it would not be amiss to give him great credit as the first physician to put to clinical use the new knowledge developed by physiologists in those days. In 1867, Adam Politzer[2] described his case as "*Symptome der Ménière' schen Erkrankungsform*" or "*Symptome der Ménièreschen Krankheitsform*" in *Archiev für Ohrenheilkunde*. In 1902, Politzer[3] made the following comment on this disease: The term "Ménière's disease," which was originally applied to sudden deafness, was later used in a broader sense and was applied to various diseases of the ear and central nervous system running their course with attacks of dizziness. This generalization brought about a certain amount of confusion, so that we are now very often satisfied with the diagnosis Ménière's disease, Ménière's dizziness, and Ménière's symptoms without taking into consideration the anatomical seat of the affection giving rise to the combination of symptoms. In his description we can learn what was the understanding of physicians on this disease in those days. In 1838, Hallpike and Cairns[4] from London and Yamakawa[5] from Osaka discovered independently the pathologic findings in definitive cases of this disease. Since then, many additional cases have been followed. In most cases, but not all, gross dilatation of the endolymphatic system without inflammatory changes was reported. Since the first discoveries by Hallpike, Cairns and Yamakawa, the term "Ménière's disease" seemed to become more common than the term "Ménière's syndrome". In 1947, Williams[6] thought that the term "Ménière's disease" had become confusing and should be dropped because it had been connected with so many different pathologic entities. He proposed the term "endolymphatic hydrops (EH)" as a more accurately descriptive one for Ménière's disease. The term "Ménière's disease," however, was so widely prevalent that his proposal has not been generally accepted. Thus the term "Ménière's disease" remains in its obscurity.

In order to find a mutually agreeable concept of Ménière's disease, in this chapter the author would like to put in order the current concept supported by Ménière's disease researchers.

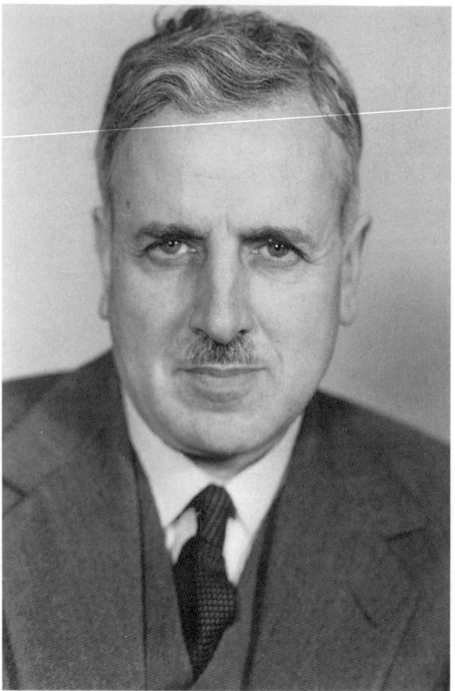

Fig. 1.1. Charles Skinner Hallpike (1900–1979)

The Current Concept of Ménière's Disease

There have been several large-scale attempts to define Ménière's disease precisely. In 1972 the Subcommittee on Equilibrium and Its Measurement of the American Academy of Ophthalmology and Otolaryngology (AAOO) defined Ménière's disease as a disease of deafness, vertigo, and usually tinnitus having as its pathologic correlate hydropic distention of the endolymphatic system. The committee also defined cochlear Ménière's disease and vestibular Ménière's disease as subvarieties of Ménière's disease[7]. In 1980 the Committee on Terminology and Definition proposed the following concept at the post-conference symposium of the First International Symposium on Pathogenesis, Diagnosis and Treatment of Ménière's Disease; Ménière's disease is a clinical entity. The etiology is unknown. All three symptoms must be present for the clinical diagnosis of Ménière's disease. Ménière's disease may have as its pathologic correlate hydropic distention of the membranous labyrinth. However, EH is a pathologic diagnosis; therefore, Ménière's disease should not be called EH unless pathology is proven. In 1985 the Committee on Hearing and Equilibrium of the American Academy of Otolaryngology—Head and Neck Surgery (AAO-HNS)—agreed to be restrictive and to include only those cases with the full complement of classic symptoms and findings of the disease presumed to result from idiopathic EH (IEH). The terms "cochlear" or "vestibular" Ménière's disease were excluded from Ménière's disease because of an absence of

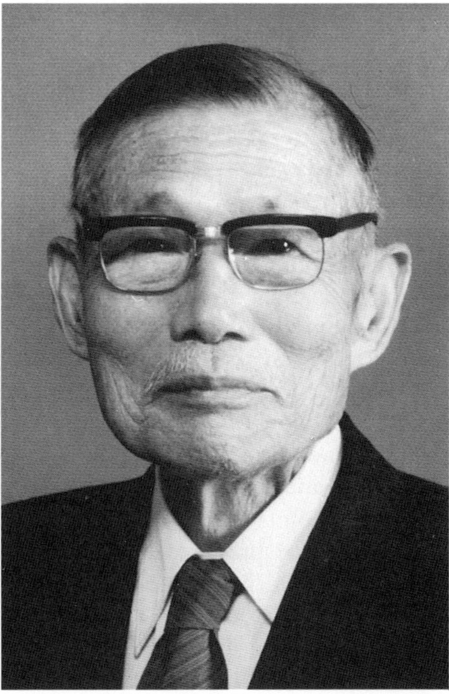

Fig. 1.2. Kyoshiro Yamakawa (1892–1980)

documentation that these variants are based on the same pathologic disorder as Ménière's disease[8].

For the past 10 years, I have made a survey of the current concept of Ménière's disease. Though it is difficult to categorize clearly, the concepts of Ménière's disease could be classified as 3 types: (1) that synonymous with Ménière's syndrome or Ménière's syndrome with unknown etiology, (2) a nosologic entity defined by characteristic clinical pictures, and (3) that synonymous with IEH.

Ménière's Syndrome or Ménière's Syndrome with Unknown Etiology

This concept is similar to that indicating a nosologic entity characterized by specific symptoms. However, most researchers who support this concept agree that the term "Ménière's syndrome" is better than the term "Ménière's disease." A.J. Duvall III (1980, personal communication) clearly states his personal opinion of the definition of Ménière's disease. He prefers the term "Ménière's syndrome" to "Ménière's disease." Since Ménière's disease is a symptom complex, the etiology of this disease is not necessarily unknown. If Ménière's disease is defined as an unknown etiological disease, the name will disappear when all etiologies have been discovered. According to Duvall, his preferred term will not disappear if all etiologies are revealed, because it will still be a symptom-complex diagnosis. This is the reason why Duvall prefers the use of syndrome to disease. Per-G. Lundquist (1980, personal communication) also states that "Ménière's syndrome" is a more suitable term even in situations where we have excluded all other known diseases.

In 1970, Jongkees [9] stated that Ménière's disease is an idiopathic syndrome; if other problems (otitis, otosclerosis, mumps, high blood pressure, diabetes, syphilis, etc.) complicate the clinical picture, it is not wise to call these cases, which are probably secondary reactions, the primary ailment—Ménière's disease. Though he wrote in his paper that Ménière's disease is an idiopathic syndrome, he had no intention of adopting the term "idiopathic Ménière's syndrome" as a substitute for "Ménière's disease" because he wanted to avoid complications by introducing new terms as long as the term "Ménière's disease" is widely prevalent in the world. J. Helms (1980, personal communication) defines Ménière's disease as symptomatic, and thinks the term "Ménière's syndrome" is more precise than "Ménière's disease." However, he uses the term "Ménière's disease" because this term is generally accepted. C. Angerborg, D.A. Dolowitz, and R. Haye (1980, personal communication) think similarly. R. Hinchcliffe (1980, personal communication) defines Ménière's disease symptomatic and prefers the term "Ménière's disorder" rather than "Ménière's disease." He points out, however, that there is a problem in requiring all three symptoms to be present before one can diagnose Ménière's disorder, especially in those cases which are in the initial stages. His concept seems to be close to that of researchers who use the term synonymous with IEH. J.A. Hilger stated in a summary of the International Symposium on Ménière's Syndrome, which was organized by H.L. Williams in 1968, that "Ménière's syndrome" is the proper terminology rather than "Ménière's disease." This is not a specific disease, but a syndrome caused by a number of different pathological processes which tend to result in an increase in the endolymphatic pressure. In 1980, he wrote to me that in the years since the International Symposium, he had not seen or heard anything that added materially to the fundamental issue.

Symptomatically Defined Nosologic Entity

In this concept Ménière's disease is thought not to be a symptom complex but a clinical and nosologic entity. According to Pfaltz[10], Ménière's disease is a nosologic entity, characterized by tinnitus, fluctuating hearing loss, and repeated attacks of vertigo. Although there may be some histopathologic and experimental evidence supporting the hypothetic existence of an atypic cochlear and vestibular form of Ménière's disease, he insists that we must strictly reject this erroneous subdivision, i.e., the division into subvarieties from a clinical point of view. He explains why we should stick to the full complement of classic symptoms as follows: If we accept the existence of subgroups of Ménière's disease, lacking the classical triad of symptoms, the whole system of classification will get out of order and control, and we shall never be able to get an acceptable definition of this disease. U. Fisch, A. Meyer zum Gottesberge, W.J. Oosterveld, W.L. Meyerhoff, G. Zechner, and K. Janke (1980, personal communications) accept a similar concept. W.L. Meyerhoff (1980, personal communication) wrote to me that his concept is contrary to the thoughts of the late H. Williams and that they spent many hours debating the subject and could never reach an agreement. Meyerhoff, however, had made presumptive diagnoses of cochlear Ménière's disease and vestibular Ménière's disease. U. Fisch (1980, personal communication) uses the term "vestibular hydrops" or "cochlear hydrops" instead of the subvarieties of Ménière's disease. In his case, the term "cochlear" or "vestibular hydrops" is a purely clinical definition and does not mean a pathological finding.

Synonymous with IEH

Some researchers think that the use of "Ménière's disease" should be restricted to IEH with a full complement of classic symptoms, but others do not insist on the this limitation, B. McCabe's concept of Ménière's disease is quite clear and is written in the report of the 1972 AAOO criteria[7]. Another opinion of his (1980, personal communication) is as follows: The EH must be idiopathic or it is not Ménière's disease, but secondary to another cause. We cannot see the scala media in the live patient, but we can rather safely infer that hydrops exists through the results of such tests as glycerol and urea. If IEH is found to exist in a patient, the diagnosis of Ménière's disease would be made irrespective of the symptoms. If there are discrepancies between the symptomatologic and pathological findings, it would be imperative to go with the pathologic findings and use that diagnosis. For M. Portmann (1980, personal communication) Ménière's disease corresponds to IEH and nothing else. EH can be diagnosed when there are findings of crisis, fluctuant hearing loss, and when improvement is provided by diuretics or glycerol. If IEH is found without a typical clinical syndrome, the case is called Ménière's disease (not typical Ménière's disease) anyway. M.R. Dix, M. Arslan, and D.E. Brackmann (1980, personal communication) think similarly. D.E. Brackmann recognizes the possibility of the existence of undetectable hydrops on histopathological study of Ménière's disease, since it may be reversible. R. Gussen (1980, personal communication) also thinks that there may be patients with a vestibular aqueduct—endolymphatic sac size that is adequate for function if it is not called upon to do too much, but the system might fail physiologically if too much effort is required of it. In such cases, there might be symptoms during life which, in death, leave only the appearance, histologically, of a normal system.

In 1983, Schuknecht[11] defined Ménière's disease as a clinical term for idiopathic symptomatic EH. Ménière's disease is classified as "typical Ménière's disease" and "atypical Ménière's disease." The latter is also classified as "auditory Ménière's disease," "vestibular Ménière's disease," and "drop-attack Ménière's disease." Delayed hydrops is excluded from Ménière's disease. According to I. Klockhoff (1980, personal communication), a positive response to osmotic expanders, such as glycerol, justify the diagnosis of Ménière's disease even if there is no vertigo present. On the other hand, when the initial symptom is episodic vertigo, the diagnosis of Ménière's disease cannot be established until hearing symptoms appear. H.O. Baber (1980, personal communication) claims that he prefers to use terminology which specifies pathology wherever possible. At times, this is not practical where eponymous diagnostic terms are firmly fixed in the literature through long usage. In his view, "hydrops" is the preferred term to be used wherever possible. Where the symptoms and signs are cochlear only, the term would be "cochlear hydrops."

However, he does not believe one can diagnose vestibular hydrops at all since histological evidence for this diagnosis is poor. For the latter cases, he proposes the term "recurrent vestibulopathy."

B.R. Alford (1980, personal communication) supports the 1972 AAOO criteria [7] for the definition of Ménière's disease. W. House, M.M. Paparella, R.J. Wiet, A.W. Morrison, L. Naftalin, M.S. Harrison, M.L. Lawrence, and H. Silverstein (1980, personal communication) for the most part do so as well. Most of them think that they can diagnose EH clinically. There have been, they believe, many post-mortem examinations of patients that have shown classical EH, with certain clinical symptoms, which make the diagnosis and terminology quite clear.

Proposal for Standardized Concept of Ménière's Disease

When we take a general view of the above survey, it appears that researchers who support the term (idiopathic) "Ménière's syndrome", are few but scattered throughout the world. They adopt this term as referred to because of our current lack of knowledge on this symptom complex. Researchers who support the clinical nosological entity, are chiefly seen on the European continent and those who support the pathological entity are in the United Kingdom and on the American continent. This tendency seems to me to be due to the fact that autopsy cases of Ménière's disease, which revealed EH, were found first in the United Kingdom and then many cases followed in the United States, while autopsy cases which had a discrepancy between pathological and clinical findings were mainly reported from Europe.

At this point, I would like to discuss the discrepancies which make it questionable that the pathological correlate of Ménière's disease is IEH. One type of discrepancy is Ménière's disease which doesn't show EH, i.e. 2 cases reported by Berggren[12] and one case by Arnvig[13]. A case of a 50-year-old male reported by Berggren didn't show EH although he complained of vertigo and deafness. Another case, a 40-year-old female, also showed normal histology in the labyrinth. For the former case, however, clinical description was too poor to diagnose Ménière's disease, and the latter was a case of central vestibular disorder, according to Berggren. A case of a 76-year-old female reported by Arnvig seems to be similar to one of Schuknecht's with endolymphatic collapse [14]. In 1960, Wustrow and Borkowsky [15] cited some autopsy cases of Ménière's disease (syndrome) which showed normal histology in the labyrinth. Most of the cases, however, were those reported before Hallpike, Cairns and Yamakawa found EH in Ménière's disease. It is uncertain if Wustrow and Borkowsky's cases were Ménière's disease or not. Of course, as previously mentioned reasonable interpretations are given to Ménière's disease with normal histology by Gussen, Brackmann, and others. Another type of discrepancy is in asymptomatic cases with histologic evidence of EH such as those of Rollins [16]. For these cases, Schuknecht[11] gave an excellent explanation when he classified these cases as "asymptomatic EH". In my opinion, one must be careful to recognize the absence of symptoms of Ménière's disease. It has been our experience that patients with Ménière's disease are often unaware of fluctuant hearing loss even though it has been proven by repeated audiometries. We also know well that some subjects complain of dizziness or a floating sensation and not of vertigo while their ears are being irrigated. It is nearly impossible to definitely state the absence of cochlear and/or vestibular symptoms during life when reviewing autopsy cases. Moreover, autopsy cases such as Arnvig's and Bergrren's are exception- less than 5% of those had Ménière's disease. All other reported autopsy cases of Ménière's disease in the literature show distention of the Reissner's membrane. Therefore, EH can be considered to be a common pathological finding in Ménière's disease. Symptoms seen in Ménière's disease may be the result of an unknown etiologic disease process that produces EH and/or EH itself.

As M.M. Paparella(1980) writes, there are many variants of Ménière's disease so that they often do not present with the classical picture. Nevertheless, one makes a diagnosis based on clinical findings and still, primarily, on information derived from the medical history. W.J. Oostrveld(1980) also complains that to make a diagnosis on the symptoms and signs only with complete uncertainty of what is really going on, makes us very uncomfortable. It is preferable to use terminology which specifies the pathology in order to provide a common ground for management of the disease. If the diagnosis of the disease is restricted to cases with a full complement of classic symptoms, then the diagnosis of Ménière's disease at its incipient stage is impossible, as most researchers have been mentioned. Physicians who would normally treat the disease may not be able to cope with it. Actually, even physicians who use the term "Ménière's disease" restrictively to cases with classic symptoms, frequently diagnose incipient monosymptomatic cases as Ménière's disease especially when the initial symptom is fluctuant hearing loss. Certainly, the disgnosis of EH is said to be impossible or difficult during life. However, most physicians believe that the continued use of the temporal bones of patients with Ménière's disease will add to their competency in making correct diagnosis during life.

Based upon the various views shown in this survey and the above considerations, I would like to define Ménière's disease as a disease with the full complement of the classic triad of symptoms and with findings presumed to be related to IEH (in a few cases we might see a normal endolymphatic system). This concept is almost the same as that proposed in 1972 AAOO and 1985 AAO-HNS criteria [7, 8]. However, cochlear Ménière's disease or Ménière's disease without vertigo (cases in which patients are unaware of vestibular symptoms may be included), is a subvariety of Ménière's disease since EH is readily identified by a glycerol test, and is proved in autopsy cases [17–20]. According to Kitahara [21], 80% of cochlear Ménière's disease proceeds to Ménière's disease in an average of 3 years. This fact can also be part of the evidence supporting the idea that cochlear Ménière's disease is an incipient Ménière's disease. This is, we believe, the most currently accepted or acceptable concept of Ménière's disease. Since no histopathological evidence on vestibular Ménière's disease is available, vestibular Ménière's disease should be excluded from the subvarities. Furthermore, only 21% of vestibular Ménière's disease proceeded to Ménière's disease in approximately 5 years[21]. Vestibular Ménière's disease may not be regarded as an early stage of Ménière's disease.

Table 1.1. Diagnostic criteria for Ménière's disease (Ménière's Disease Research Committee, 1974)

1. Repeated attacks of vertigo
   a Episodes of dizziness without specific cause which are accompanied by nausea or vomiting, lasting several minutes to several hours
   b There may be some episodes of non-whirling dizziness included in the series of vertigo
   c A mixed type of spontaneous nystagmus (horizontal and rotatory) is observed in most cases during attacks
   d In cases with a single first attack, differential diagnosis with sudden sensorineural deafness is especially important
2. Fluctuating cochlear symptoms
   a Tinnitus and/or hearing loss often fluctuate synchronously with the vertiginous attacks
   b Many patients complain of fullness in the ear and hypersensitivity to intense sound in the affected ear
   c The hearing tests reveal a marked fluctuation of the threshold of hearing in the low and middle tone range; loudness recruitment will be observed; usually only one ear is affected, however, bilateral involvement is not rare
3. Exclusion of central nervous system involvement, VIIIth nerve tumor and other cochleovestibular disease. To exclude these other disorders, a thorough history, neurological examination, and specific clinical examinations including equilibrium function tests and audiological tests must be performed; at times it is necessary to follow the patient's course in order to obtain the required chronological information necessary for establishing the correct diagnosis

Diagnostic criteria
I. Conformable to conditions 1–3: diagnosis is definite
II. Conformable to conditions 1 and 3, or 2 and 3: diagnosis is suspicious or uncertain

Diagnostic Criteria for Ménière's Disease

In 1978, the Ménière's Disease Research Committee proposed the diagnostic criteria for Ménière's disease as shown in Table 1.1. This diagnostic criteria is not so doctrinary that this disease is strictly restricted to cases with the full complement of the classic triad. For example, repeated attacks of vertigo are one of important symptoms for diagnosing Ménière's disease. According to this idea, Ménière's disease is not diagnosed for any patient who has had one attack only. In our criteria, even in cases with a single attack, a diagnosis of Ménière's disease is given if it is differentiated from sudden deafness. Our committee tried to see the whole picture of Ménière's disease, including initial and advanced stages of the disease. In order to exclude central nervous system involvement, such as acoustic neurinomas and other cochleovestibular disorders, neurological examinations have been carried out intensively. Later, CT Scan and NMR were introduced and the exclusion of such diseases became very precise. In 1988, the Vestibular Disorders Research Committee presented the guidelines for the procedure and clinical significance in the use of the Glycerol Test, Furosemide Test, and the ECohG in detecting EH. A diagnosis of Ménière's disease which has been made based on clinical findings and still, primarily, on information derived from the medical history, is expected to be

Table 1.2. Diagnostic criteria for Ménière's disease with bilateral fluctuant hearing loss (Vestibular Disorders Research Committee, 1988)

1. Repeated attacks of vertigo
   a Dizzy spells without specific cause which are accompanied by nausea or vomiting lasting several minutes to several hours
   b There may be some episodes of nonwhirling dizziness included in the series of vertigo
   c In cases with a single first attack, differential diagnosis with sudden sensorineural deafness is especially important
2. Fluctuant cochlear symptoms in bilateral ears
   a Tinnitus and/or hearing loss often show fluctuation synchronous with the vertiginous attacks
   b Many patients complain of fullness in the ear and hypersensitivity to intense sound
   c Cochlear symptoms appear simultaneously or alternately in both ears. Since patients who suffer from bilateral involvement are often unaware of a slight deafness and/or tinnitus in the contralateral ear, it is necessary to confirm the deafness in both ears by means of frequent audiometry or glycerol tests
   d The hearing test reveal a marked fluctuation of the threshold of hearing in the low and middle tone range; recruitment of loudness will be observed
3. Exclusion of central nervous system involvement, VIIIth nerve tumor and other cochleovestibular disease

Diagnostic criteria

I. Conformable to conditions 1–3: diagnosis is definite

II. In the following cases conformable to condition 3: diagnosis is suspicious or uncertain
   a Ménière's disease with nonfluctuant tinnitus and/or hearing loss in the contralateral ear
   b Cases with recurrent attacks of vertigo and hearing loss and/or tinnitus in both ears
   c Cases with hearing loss and/or tinnitus in both ears and these cochlear symptoms fluctuating at least in one ear.

actively verified by means of the above techniques. In 1988, the diagnostic criteria for Ménière's disease with bilateral fluctuant hearing loss was also proposed by our committee (Table 1.2). The first nation-wide survey concerning the bilaterality of this disease was carried out at that time (see Chap 2).

It is necessary to obtain mutually agreeable diagnostic criteria for Ménière's disease so that a common ground for management of this disease is provided and so that everyone will be able to compare similar manifestations. Diagnostic criteria will be determined by the concept of the disease. However, when the criteria is made too rigid in order to get "pure" Ménière's disease, many potential cases of Ménière's disease will be dropped and we will fail to see the whole picture of this disease. When the criteria is made too loose, patients with diseases other than Ménière's disease will be diagnosed as having Ménière's disease. It is necessary to improve the diagnostic criteria according to the developments in science. In formulating better and more reasonable clinical criteria, one should always bear all of these ideas in mind.

Acknowledgment. The author would like to express his heartfelt appreciation and gratitude to researchers for sharing their conceptions of Ménière's disease as quoted in the text.

References

1. Ménière P (1861) Maladie de l'oreille interne offarnt les symptomes de la congestion cerebrate apoplectiforme. Gaz Med Paris 3:88
2. Politzer A (1867) Über Lasion des Labyrinthes. Arch Ohrenheilk 2:88–99
3. Politzer A (1902) A textbook of the diseases of the ear. Tindall and Cox Bailliere
4. Hallpike CS, Cairns H (1938) Observations on the pathology of Ménière's syndrome. J Laryngol Otol 53:625–655
5. Yamakawa K (1938) Über die pathologische Veränderung bei einem Ménière-Kranken. J Otolaryngol Jpn 44:2310–2312
6. Williams HL (1947) The present status of the diagnosis and treatment of endolymphatic hydrops. Ann Otol Rhinol Laryngol 54:614–646
7. Alford BR (1972) Report of subcommittee on equilibrium and its measurement. Trans Pa Acad Opthalmol Otolaryngol 76:1462–1464
8. Pearson BW, Brackmann DE (1985) Committee on hearing and equilibrium guidelines for reporting treatment results in Ménière's disease. Otolaryngol Head Neck Surg 93: 579–582
9. Jongkees LBW (1979) Some remarks on Ménière's disease. J Otorhinolaryngol Relat Spec 42:1–5
10. Pfaltz CR (1986) A tentative retro-and prospective outline. In: Pfaltz CR (ed) Controversial aspects of Ménière's disease. Georg Thieme, Stuttgart, pp 138–147
11. Schuknecht HF, Gulya AJ (1983) Endolymphatic hydrops. An overview and classification. Ann Otol Rhinol Laryngol 92:1–20
12. Berggren S (1949) Histological investigation of three cases with Ménière's syndrome. Acta Otolaryngol (Stockh) 37:30–36
13. Arnvig J (1947) Histological findings in a case of Ménière's disease with remarks on the pathologic anatomical basis of this lesion. Acta Otolaryngol (Stockh) 35:453–466
14. Schuknecht HF (1962) Further observation on the pathology of Ménière's disease. Ann Otol Rhinol Laryngol 71:1039–1053
15. Wustrow F, Borkowsky B (1960) Ergebnisse nach konservation und chirurgischen Behandlungsmethoden sowie kritische Betrachtungen zur Pathogenese des Morbus Ménière. Z Laryngol 39:133–152
16. Rollins H (1940) Zur Kenntnis des labyrinth. Hydrops und des durch ihn bedingten Ménière. HNO 31:73–109
17. Lindsay JR (1946) Labyrinthine dropsy. Laryngoscope 56:315–341
18. Lindsay JR, Schulthess G (1958) An unusual case of labyrinthine hydrops. Acta Otolaryngol (Stockh) 49:315–324
19. Altmann F, Kornfeld M (1965) Histological studies of Ménière's disease. Ann Otol Rhinol Laryngol 74:915–943
20. Kohut RI, Lindsay JR (1972) Pathologic changes in idiopathic labyrinthine hydrops. Acta Otolaryngol (Stockh) 73:402–412
21. Kitahara M, Takeda T, Yazawa Y, Matsubara H, Kitano H (1984) Pathophysiology of Ménière's Disease and Its Subvarieties. Acta Otolaryngol [Suppl] (Stockh) 406:52–55

CHAPTER 2

Ménière's Disease with Bilateral Fluctuant Hearing Loss

Masaaki Kitahara, Hiroya Kitano, and Mikio Suzuki

Although bilateral involvement of Ménière's disease can produce deafness in both ears, actually little attention had been directed to this involvement. In 1959, Jongkees[1] reported the high incidence involving the second ear in order to warn of a dangerous trend toward using destructive procedures in the treatment of this disease at that time. Since then, several reports concerning the bilateral aspects of this disease have appeared [2–8]. However, the lack of mutually agreeable diagnostic criteria for making these reports and the differences in Ménière's disease characteristics of patients among institutes makes it difficult to establish definitive interpretations. In 1988, the Vestibular Disorder Research Committee made a survey among 15 committee member institutes using the same diagnostic criteria of bilateral involvement of Ménière's disease. Based on the results obtained, the incidence and characteristics of bilateral involvement in Ménière's disease will be discussed in this chapter.

Methods and Materials

The diagnostic criteria of Ménière's disease and Ménière's disease with bilateral fluctuant hearing loss are shown in Chap. 1 (Tables 1.1, 1.2). In this study, unilateral Ménière's disease refers to the condition in which the cochlear symptom is limited to one ear. The study is based on 480 cases of Ménière's disease from 15 committee member institutes between April 1, 1988 and September 30, 1988. A total of 201 cases (91 male, 110 female) showed normal hearing in the second ear (unilateral Ménière's disease or cases with unilateral involvement). In 135 cases (58 male, 77 female), fluctuant cochlear symptoms in the second ear were present (Ménière's disease with bilateral fluctuant hearing loss or bilateral involvement). Another 10 cases (3 male, 7 female) showed progressive hearing loss in the second ear (Ménière's disease with progressive sensorineural hearing loss). The types of hearing loss in the second ear of the remaining 134 cases were not clear.

The following items were checked for each of the Ménière's disease patients:

1. Level of hearing in both ears
2. Types of hearing in the second ear—fluctuant sensorineural hearing loss, fluctuant tinnitus, progressive sensorineural hearing loss, other types of sensorineural hearing loss, and others

3. Disturbance of equilibrium function—positive Romberg or ataxic gait, positive spontaneous nystagmus or positional nystagmus, and an abnormal caloric test
4. Course of the disease—duration of disease, number of attacks since the disease began, regular recurrence, irregular recurrence, cluster attacks, sporadic attacks, evolvement of attacks from vertigo to continuous dizziness, and physicians' judgments on the general course of the disease (improvement, fluctuation, fixation, or worsening)
5. Physician's evaluation—if an intractable type, why?

Results

The average age at the onset of unilateral Ménière's disease was shown to be 42.1 years and that of Ménière's disease with bilateral fluctuant hearing loss, 46.2 years (Fig. 2.1). Figure 2.2 shows duration of the disease from the time of onset of initial

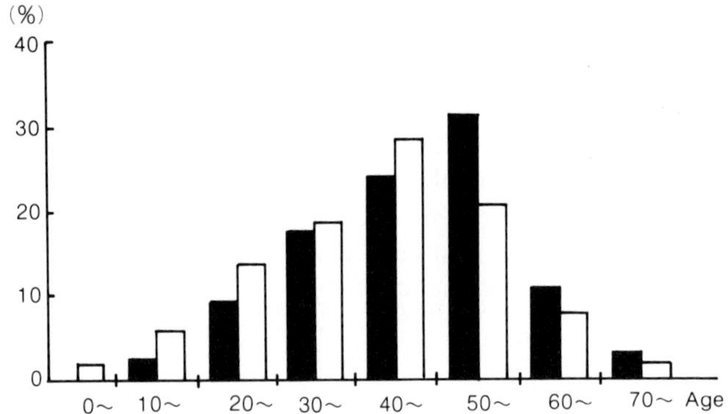

Fig. 2.1. Distribution of age (years) at onset of Ménière's disease. *white column*, unilateral involvement; *black column*, bilateral involvement

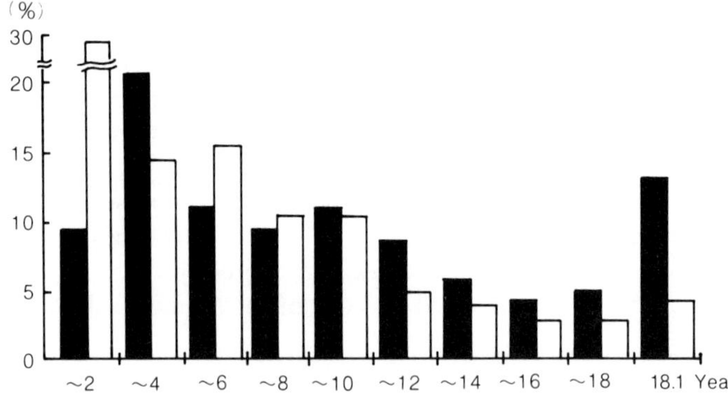

Fig. 2.2. Distribution of duration of Ménière's disease. *white column*, unilateral involvement; *black column*, bilateral involvement

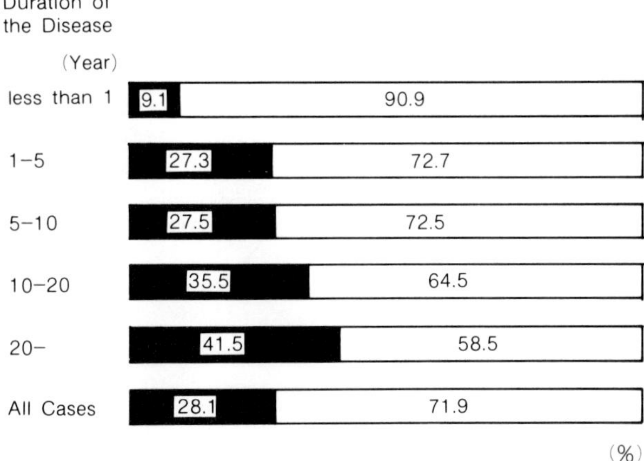

Fig. 2.3. Percentage of bilateral involvement among all investigated cases ($n = 480$) of Ménière's disease in each period of duration. *white column*, unilateral involvement; *black column*, bilateral involvement

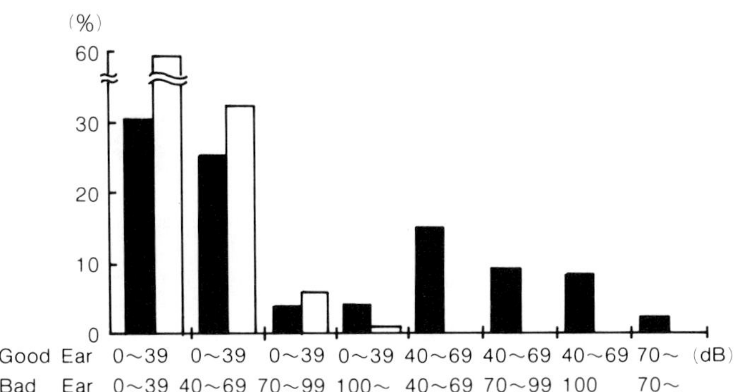

Fig. 2.4. Level of hearing in both ears in cases of Ménière's disease. *white column*, unilateral involvement; *black column*, bilateral involvement

symptoms to the time of the survey. The average duration of the disease was 6.5 years in unilateral involvement and 9.9 years in bilateral involvement. The duration of the disease in cases of bilateral involvement was significantly longer than that in unilateral involvement. Figure 2.3 shows the ratio of cases with bilateral involvement among all investigated cases of Ménière's disease in each period of duration. Bilateral involvement was found in 28% or 135 out of the 480 cases of Ménière's disease. Cases with bilateral involvement accounted for 41% of the patients who had had the disease for 20 years or more, but only 9% of the patients who had had the disease for 1 year or less.

Figure 2.4 compares the levels of hearing in both ears in cases of Ménière's disease with unilateral and bilateral involvements. Even when cases were limited to those in which the level of hearing was 0–39 dB in the good ear, the level of hearing in

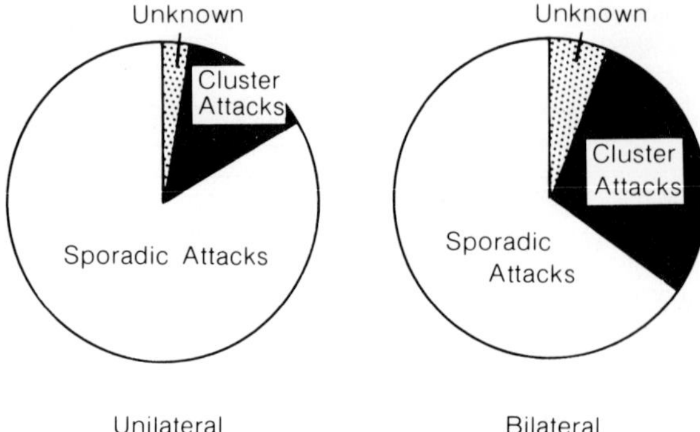

Fig. 2.5. Patterns of attack of Ménière's disease

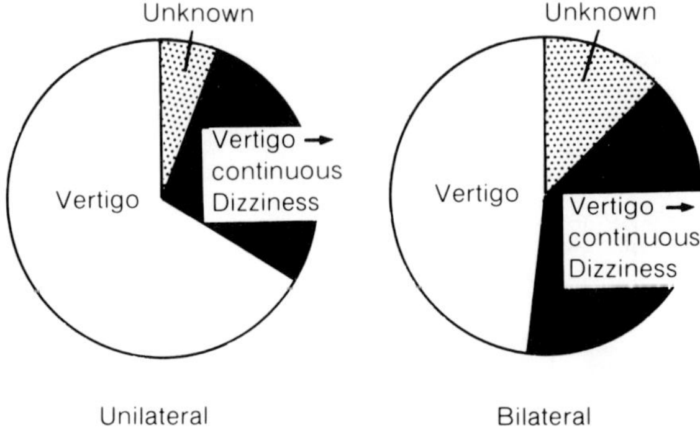

Fig. 2.6. Evolvement of attacks from vertigo to continuous dizziness in cases of Ménière's disease

the bad ear seemed to be worse in cases with bilateral involvement than in those with unilateral involvement. In both cases, as Figures 2.5 and 2.6 show, sporadic attacks were more frequently observed than cluster attacks. Cluster attacks, however, were more frequently observed in cases with bilateral involvement. Similarly, attacks evolved from vertigo to continuous dizziness more frequently in cases with bilateral involvement. In a comparison of physicians' evaluations of the course of the disease (Table 2.1), most felt that in unilateral cases the condition had been improved. In cases with bilateral involvement, however, most had fluctuated or fixed at a worsened condition. The average frequency of attacks of vertigo was 6.5 times per year in unilateral cases and 3.5 times per year in bilateral cases.

Table 2.2 shows the reasons the physicians gave for recognizing their patients' Ménière's disease as intractable. In cases with bilateral involvement, 43% (58 out of 135 cases) were considered to be intractable by their physicians. On the other hand, only 5% (10 out of 201 cases) with unilateral involvement were described as intractable. This decision was due to disequilibrium in 26% of the cases with

Table 2.1. Physicians' evaluation of the course of the disease in their Ménière's patients

Course	Unilateral involvement (%)	Bilateral involvement (%)
Improved	49	28
Fluctuated	28	42
Stabilized	15	21
Worse	4	4
Unknown	4	5

Table 2.2. Reasons the physicians recognized the disease in some of their Ménière's patients as being intractable

Reason	Unilateral involvement (%)	Bilateral involvement (%)
Deafness	7	28
Disequilibrium	26	9
Long Duration	22	12
Progressiveness	15	7
Bilateral Deafness	—	33
Psychological	4	5
Problems	15	3
Social Problems	11	3
Others		

unilateral involvement. In contrast, in 61% of the cases with bilateral involvement, it was due to bilateral hearing loss.

Ménière's disease with progressive hearing loss in the second ear was observed in approximately 2% or 10 out of 480 cases. The average duration was 13.2 years, average age at onset of the disease was 39.5 years, and average frequency of attacks was 2.2 times per year.

Discussion

The term "Ménière's disease" is usually limited to patients with trial symptoms, i.e., vertigo, deafness, and tinnitus. When using the term "bilateral Ménière's disease" according to this concept, both ears must be responsible either simultaneously or alternately for the occurrence of vertigo as well as for cochlear symptoms. It is conceivable that even though both ears show fluctuant hearing loss the vertigo attacks or repetitive fluctuant vestibular dysfunctions may be caused by the ear of one and the same side only. The term "bilateral Ménière's disease" seems to be unsuitable in this case. Though it is rather difficult for patients to be aware of a mild or slight hearing deficiency or tinnitus in the second ear, it is possible to reveal fluctuant hearing loss with frequent monitoring by audiometry or glycerol tests. It is quite difficult, however, to prove that both ears are responsible either simultaneously or alternately for vertiginous attacks. Even when using equilibrium testing to evaluate the vestibular system, the test results do not accurately indicate which side, if it is only one side, or whether both sides are responsible. In this respect, the term "bilateral Ménière's disease" can be applied only to those rare cases where both ears are incidentally proven to be responsible for the vertiginous attacks. Based on these considerations, the term "Ménière's disease with bilateral fluctuant hearing loss" was adopted instead of the term "bilateral Ménière's disease." The term "bilateral Ménière's disease" can be substituted for the former if the substitution is clearly stated.

The incidence of cases with bilateral involvement was 28% and increased with the duration of the disease. The percentage increased from 9% (at less than 1 year) to 41% when the duration of the disease was more than 20 years. A rate of approximately 30%, which came from multiple institutes with the same diagnostic criteria, is considered to be reasonable although it may vary according to region, race, and time of survey. This tendency was similar in most reports [2, 4, 6, 7] in the past few years. This incidence with bilateral involvement (28%) is also very close to that of bilateral endolymphatic hydrops found in our review of the literature on 72 temporal bone autopsy cases of Ménière's disease[4, 9]. These facts increase the veracity of the figures of incidence of this survey.

No difference of sex distribution between the two groups was observed. The age at the onset of the disease was a little higher in cases with bilateral involvement than with unilateral involvement. The course of Ménière's disease with bilateral involvement was more severe than that with unilateral involvement; the duration was longer and attacks were likely to evolve from vertigo to continuous dizziness despite being less frequent than in unilateral involvement. In this regard, bilaterality is considered to be a distinctive marker indicating whether the disease is intractable or not. Moreover, it is also important to realize that most physicians looked upon cases with bilateral involvement as intractable because of the hearing loss being bilateral. Actually, the degree of hearing loss in the bad ear, in cases with bilateral involvement, was more severe than that in unilateral cases. At the same time, vestibular function was not as affected in bilateral cases as in unilateral cases. These findings must be taken into account when proceeding with treatment. In other words, management for an anticipated hearing loss should take precedence over disequilibrium in cases of bilateral involvement. When surgical treatment such as intramastoid drainage is selected for cases of bilateral involvement, precedence should be given to the ear in which deafness must be prevented if discrepancy for the responsibility to hearing and equilibrium exists. Administration of ototoxic drugs, which may cause hearing loss and/or disequilibrium, must be done with extreme caution.

In our survey, the second ear in 10 cases of Ménière's disease had a progressive sensorineural hearing loss. Since the duration of this type of Ménière's disease (13.2 years) was longer than that of Ménière's disease with bilateral fluctuant hearing loss (9.9 years), the former type of Ménière's disease must either be an advanced case with bilateral fluctuant hearing loss or one of a special type. In this study, we have no evidence to distinguish between them. In either case, however, this type of Ménière's disease again suggests the severity of bilateral involvement.

In this paper, the high incidence and severity of bilateral involvement have been emphasized. The question is whether or not these characteristics of bilateral involvement found in recent studies are based only on increased awareness of the possibility of bilateral involvement, earlier detection of manifestations of the disease, or longer follow-up. Is it not conceivable that the discovery of these characteristics are due to an increasing number of etiological factors which may effect bilateral involvement? Recent studies (Vestibular Disorder Research Committee) show a more frequent occurrence of Ménière's disease in females than in males. This finding coincides with the sex distribution of Ménière's disease with progressive sensorineural hearing loss and gives us a presentiment of the reality of the above hypothesis. In a previous report by one of the authors [4], it was suggested that general predisposition must be predominant over the local one in cases with bilateral involvement. It is urgent to reveal the nature of the bilaterality which makes this malady most intractable.

Acknowledgments. We are deeply grateful to our committee members for their cooperation in this study.

References

1. Jongkees LBW (1959) Vestibulogene vertigo. Ned Tijdschr Geneeskd 103:2429–2438
2. Enander A, Stahle J (1967) Hearing in Ménière's disease. Acta Otolaryngol (Stockh) 64:543–556
3. Greven AJ, Oosterveld WJ (1975) The contralateral ear in Ménière's disease. Arch Otolaryngol 101:608–612
4. Kitahara M, Matsubara H, Takeda T, Yazawa Y (1979) Bilateral Ménière's disease. Adv Otorhinolaryngol 25:117–121
5. Mizukoshi K (1979) Epidemiological survey of definite cases of Ménière's disease. Adv Otorhinolaryngol 25:106
6. Balkany TJ, Sires B, Arenberg IK (1980) Bilateral aspects of Ménière's disease. Otolaryngol Clin North Am 13:603–610
7. Paparella MM, Griebie MS (1984) Bilaterality of Ménière's disease. Acta Otolaryngol (Stockh) 97:233–237
8. Pfaltz CR (1986) A tentative retro- and prospective outline. In: Pfaltz CR (ed) Controversial aspects of Ménière's disease. Georg Thieme, Stuttgart, pp 138–147
9. Yazawa Y, Kitahara M (1990) Bilateral endolymphatic hydrops in Ménière's disease: Review of temporal bone autopsies. Ann Otol Rhinol Laryngol 99:524–528

Part II. Pathophysiology of Ménière's Disease

CHAPTER 3

The Physical Strength of the Membranous Labyrinth and Its Relation to Endolymphatic Hydrops

Tetsuo Ishii, Nobukazu Yamamoto, and Terufumi Machida

Pathological findings of Ménière's disease were first reported by Hallpike and Cairns [1]. The main finding was an enlarged endolymphatic space of the cochlear duct and saccule which was called "endolymphatic hydrops." Subsequent histopathological studies on temporal bones with Ménière's disease have confirmed the presence of endolymphatic hydrops in the cochlea and saccule, although some investigators reported enlargement of the utricle or deformity of the semicircular canal [2, 3].

The reason the endolymphatic hydrops occurred in the pars inferior of the labyrinth has not yet been thoroughly understood. Decreased absorptive function of the endolymphatic sac could influence the longitudinal flow of endolymph from cochlea to saccule, resulting in an accumulation of endolymph. The occurrence of vertigo and nystagmus was explained by the rupture of the membranous labyrinth [4]. On the other hand, the presence of hydrops was thought to create mechanical disorders in the cochlea which explain the hearing loss of Ménière's disease [5].

Endolymphatic hydrops is produced by an increase of endolymph. This volume increase could possibly be caused by high osmotic pressure in the endolymphatic space due to unknown pathological conditions. Is the volume increase localized only in the pars inferior of the labyrinth? It is a well-known fact that an endolymphatic valve exists between the utricle and the utricular duct. This valve may prevent the increased endolymph from passing to the pars superior of the labyrinth. The structure of the valve, however, seems delicate. Specifically, the utricular wall facing the tip of the valve is extremely thin (Fig. 3.1). The shift of fluid could take place through the valve.

It is possible to maintain that the increase of endolymph occurs in the entire endolymphatic space of the labyrinth. However the thickness of membranes in various parts of the labyrinth differs. Figure 3.1 shows the differences of thickness in the membranous labyrinth of the same subject. As far as histological findings are concerned, Reissner's and the saccular membranes are the thinnest. The utricular membrane of the valve portion is also thin, while membranes of other portions of the utricle and semicircular canals are thick. The thickness of these parts was measured from temporal bone sections of 10 cases. The thickness of the semicircular canal was 0.027 mm, utricular membrane 0.026, saccular membrane 0.015 and Reissner's membrane 0.014. It is speculated that the volume increase of

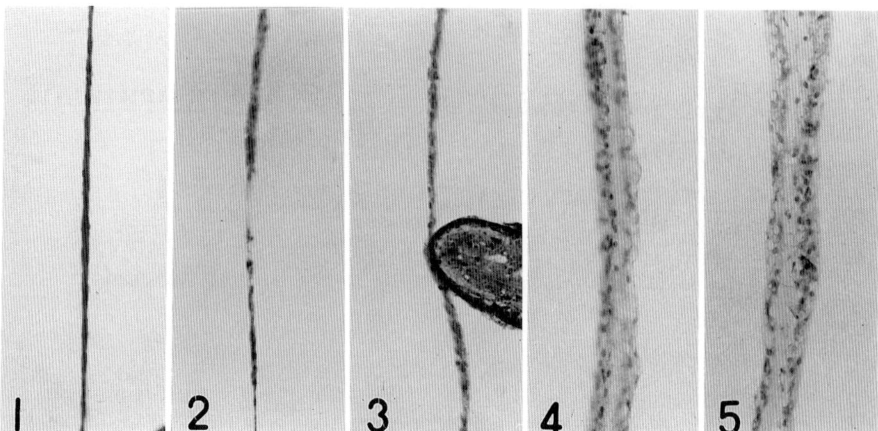

Fig. 3.1. Comparison of various parts of the human membranous labyrinth from the same individual and at the same magnification. *1*, Reissner's membrane; *2*, saccular membrane; *3*, utricular membrane facing the valve; *4*, utricular membrane; *5*, semicircular canal

endolymph in the entire labyrinth produces distension of the membranes only in the weakest parts of the labyrinth, i.e. the pars inferior.

We suspected that a thin membrane is weaker than a thick one in the labyrinth. To obtain direct evidence on the mechanical strength of membranes, a new apparatus was manufactured in our laboratory to estimate the mechanical properties of small-sized specimens [6, 7]. We studied the mechanical strength of fish, guinea pigs and human tympanic membranes [6] and membranous labyrinths [7].

Microtension Tester

A device was designed for measuring the microload (capacity: 200 gf), for observing the specimens, and for performing automatic measurements (Takachiho Seiki Co. Ltd., 1987) (Fig. 3.2). It consists of 2 adhesive grips, an electromotive power, and an analogue recording system for the load-stroke curve and digital measurements. The main system of the tension tester is shown in Figure 3.3 (a). The control unit is located on the right side and the recorder on the left side (Fig. 3.2). The mechanism of the device is shown in Fig. 3.3b. The crosshead was driven through reduction gears by the D.C. servomotor, using an A.C. 100V electric source. Its moving or tensile velocity is adjustable in the range of $0–8.33 \times 10^{-4}$ $m \cdot s^{-1}$. Its stroke (i.e., displacement) can be measured by a potentiometer, if it is within 30.0 mm. The tensile load can be measured by a load cell of a thin flexible metal sheet, if it is within 200 gf (gram force). The control unit can adjust the grip position and the tensile rate, and can detect the tensile load.

A recorder (X-Y-T recorder, Rikadenki Kogyo Co. Ltd., 1987) was also connected to the device for obtaining the load-stroke (elongation) diagrams. Before performing the tension test, the specimen was fixed on the holder (grip) with an

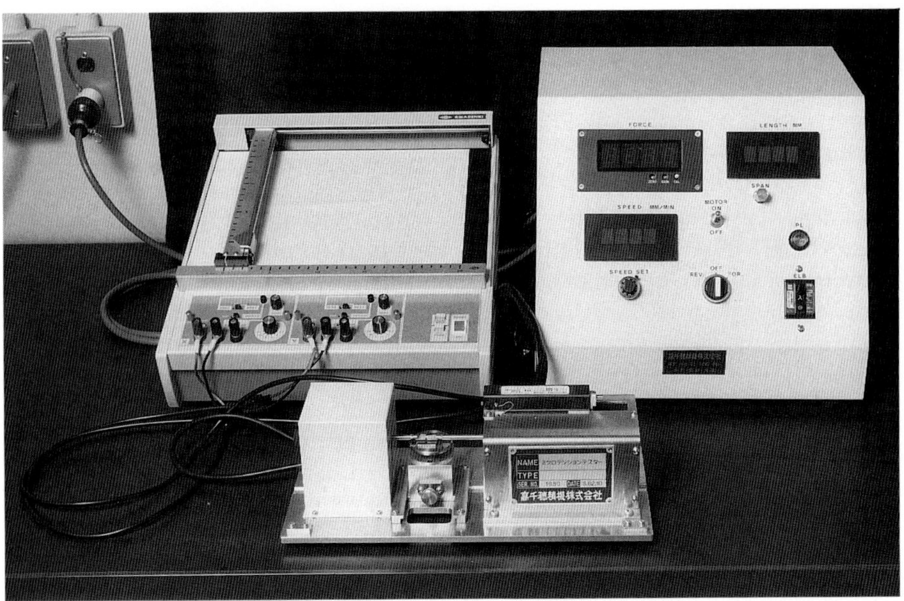

Fig. 3.2. Microtension testing device (Takachiho Seiki Co., Ltd.)

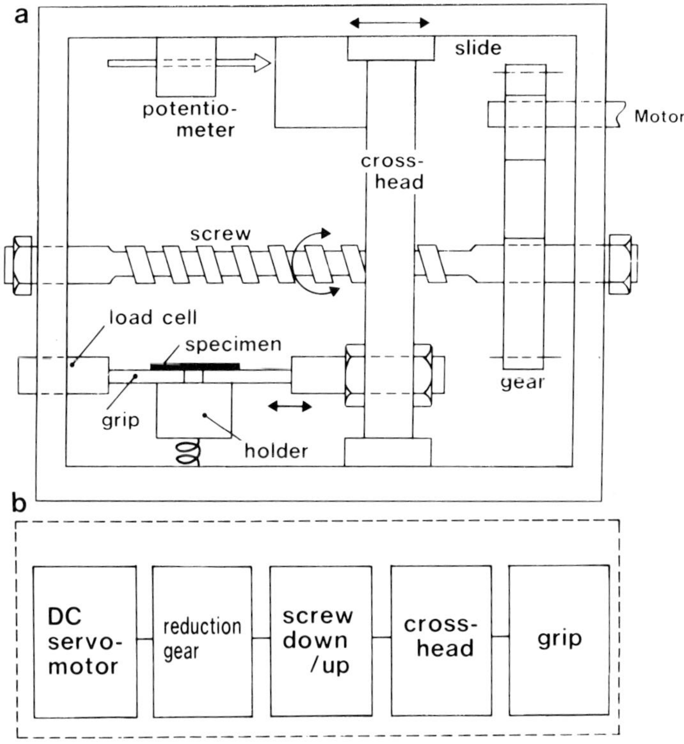

Fig. 3.3. **a** Mechanism and **b** block diagram of the microtension measuring device

adhesive tape (3M Co. Ltd.) and/or with an adhesive agent (Alon Alpha). The distance between both grips, the gauge length, is 0.3 mm.

Materials and Methods

Specimens of membranous labyrinths were obtained from the following sources [7]: 12 ears from 7 Hartley strain albino guinea pigs with body weights of 270–350 g, showing normal Preyer's reflex; 8 ears from 5 frogs (*Rana catesbeiana*); and 6 ears from 3 freshwater fish (*Carassius carassius langsdorfii*). Guinea pigs were sacrificed by intraperitoneal injection of 50 mg/kg sodium pentobarbital. The temporal bones were removed after decapitation. The semicircular canals were dissected and removed from the temporal bones.

Under ether anesthesia and injection of sodium pentobarbital, frogs were incised behind the tympanic membrane and decapitated. The semicircular canals were removed from the extirpated temporal bones. Freshwater fish were wrapped by ether-soaked linen and after being anesthetized were decapitated. Then, we dissected and removed the semicircular canals from the skulls. Tension tests for each semicircular canal were performed along the long axis at a tensile rate of $8.33 \times 10^{-4}\ \mathrm{m \cdot s^{-1}}$ at room temperature. Both fresh and formalin-fixed specimens were used for these tests.

Specimens of human membranous labyrinths from the same cadaver were obtained from both ears without any demonstrable inner ear disease. The specimens had been fixed with formalin and were examined after being washed with physiological saline solution at room temperature and at a tensile rate of $0.17 \times 10^{-4}\ \mathrm{m \cdot s^{-1}}$. Tension was applied to the semicircular canals and Reissner's membranes along the longitudinal axis. Saccular and utricular membranes were resected spherically and tension tests were performed.

Results

Semicircular Canals of Fish, Frogs and Guinea Pigs

Characteristics of the Load-Stroke (Elongation) Diagram

A steep, descending curve with one peak was observed in each case (Fig. 3.4). Each specimen showed the maximal load immediately after the terminal point of elastic deformation without ductility. The semicircular canals behaved like brittle material in the mechanical sense [7].

Force Requiring Breakdown of Formalin-fixed Specimens

Table 3.1 summarizes the measurement results. The force requiring breakdown of the semicircular canals in toto in 3 species was measured. Thickness influences

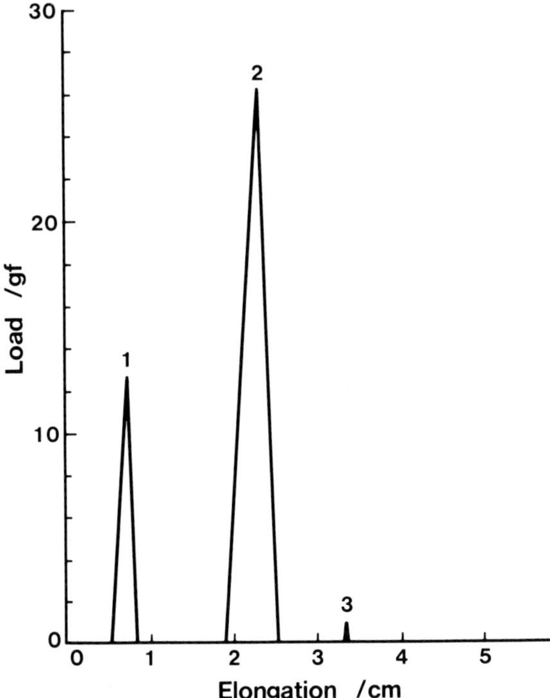

Fig. 3.4. Load—stroke (elongation) diagram of semicircular canals of 3 species, *1*, freshwater fish; *2*, frog; *3*, guinea pig

Table 3.1. Force at which breakdown of semicircular canals occurs (mean values in gram-force [gf])

	Formalin-fixed specimens	Fresh specimens
Guinea pig	0.30	0.36
Frog	23.30	31.40
Freshwater fish	20.20	18.30

Tensile rate, $8.33\text{m}^{-4}/\text{s}$

these values, because the semicircular canal of the guinea pig is much thinner than those of frogs and fish. The load required for the rupture of a guinea pig semicircular canal was 0.36gf for a fresh specimen and 0.30gf for a formalin-fixed specimen. We utilized this ratio, 0.36/0.30 (1.2), converting the value of the formalin-fixed specimen to the fresh one in human membranous labyrinths, because only formalin-fixed human labyrinths were used for this study.

As the first step of the application of the microtension tester on membranous labyrinths, tensile strength was compared among semicircular canals with different membrane thickness in mammals (guinea pig), Amphibia (frogs) and freshwater fish (Table 3.1). Although the membrane thickness of the guinea pig was not accurately measured, its strength was measured. It is known that fish lack a bony labyrinth, *but do have a thick membranous labyrinth.* Amphibia, including frogs, have a bony labyrinth, but the pars superior, which is evolutionally older in the membranous labyrinth, still has a thick membrane. This is the same order of phylogeny: during evolution, membranes of labyrinths developed but they are thought to become thinner and weaker under the protection of a bony labyrinth.

Human Membranous Labyrinth

The characteristics of load-elongation diagrams of human membranous labyrinths were similar to those of guinea pigs, frogs and fish [7]. The human membranous labyrinths were tested only with formalin-fixed materials at a tensile rate $0.17 \times 10^{-4} \mathrm{m \cdot s^{-1}}$. We tested 6 pieces of Reissner's membrane, 2 pieces of the saccular membrane, 3 pieces of the utricular membrane and 6 pieces of the semicircular canals from 2 human labyrinths. Results are shown in Table 3.2.

Conversion from Tensile Strength to Breakage Pressure

Analysis of the load-elongation diagram revealed that the human membranous labyrinth showed the same reaction as that of brittle materials. Table 3.2 shows the tensile strength of formalin-fixed specimens. These values were converted into the values for fresh specimens, according to the previously described ratio of fresh vs. formalin-fixed semicircular canals of the guinea pig. The converted values are shown in Table 3.2. This was in the same order as the membrane thickness of the labyrinth. Therefore, it suggests that the thicker the membrane is, the stronger it is. We also calculated the force requiring break-down in toto in Table 3.2. These values could be obtained from the tensile strength multiplied by the respective membrane thickness which was described previously. The modes of swelling in the membranous labyrinth are cylindrical or spherical in shape. We assumed that the mode of swelling in the membranous labyrinth is of spherical shape (Fig. 3.5). If it's action is like a hemisphere, the equation is as follows.

$$\text{Biaxial stress on top} : \sigma = \mathrm{p}\rho/2\mathrm{t} \qquad ①$$

Table 3.2. Mechanical properties of the human membranous labyrinth

	Tensile strength (gf/mm^2)		Force required for total breakdown (gf/mm) (Converted to values for fresh specimens)
	Formalin-fixed specimens ($n = 2$)	Fresh specimens (converted values*)	
Semicircular canal	150.57	165.63	4.52
Utricular membrane	82.54	90.75	2.82
Reissner's membrane	45.23	49.75	0.84
Saccular membrane	30.03	36.33	0.57

Tensile rate, $0.17 \mathrm{m}^{-4}/\mathrm{s}$
*Converted ratio, 0.36 : 0.30 (1.2)

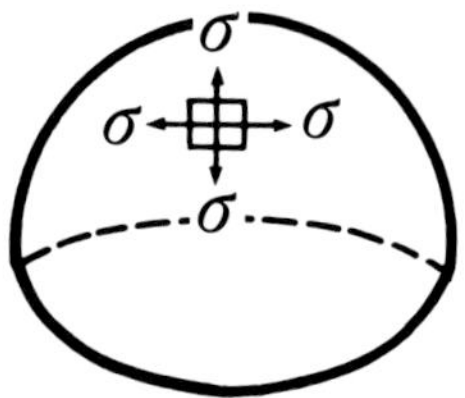

Fig. 3.5. Spherical shape demonstrating assumed mode of swelling

When the stress σ increases with pressure and reaches its maximum strength level, the material breaks.

On the other hand, the membrane has no ductility and its fracture occurs rapidly at the limit of elasticity. From this fact, it is assumed that the thickness (t) is constant during the bulging of the membrane. By using the above-mentioned considerations and equation ①, the breakage pressure (i.e., the minimal pressure for rupture of the membranous labyrinth) is computed. The radius of the curvature in these parts of the membranous labyrinth was measured from human temporal bone horizontal sections of 5 cases. Cross sections of semicircular canals and utricles appear almost round in shape, so their radii could be estimated as 0.33 and 1.68 mm, respectively. The radius of the saccule (1.13 mm) was measured from a half of the length between the anterior and posterior ends of the saccular membrane. The radius of Reissmer's membrane was calculated from a half of the distance between the upper end of the stria vascularis and the limbus spiralis. They were 0.36 mm for the basal turn and 0.48 mm for the middle turn. We know that the membrane with a larger radius of curvature is prone to rupture at a lower pressure. Thus, it is evident that membranes in the pars superior of labyrinths are mechanically stronger than those of the pars inferior.

It is well documented that the etiology of Ménière's disease is endolymphatic hydrops. This lesion develops insidiously over several years, so that it is unknown whether the tensile rate of 0.17 $m^{-4}s^{-1}$ applied in this experiment is appropriate for understanding such a lesion in the human membranous labyrinth. If the tensile rate of 0.17 $m^{-4}s^{-1}$ is an impulse for the inner ear, we must consider the rate of the effect of the strain. We reported only the real data here, because the tensile rate occurring in Ménière's disease would complicate the study. Therefore, future studies may find a smaller value for tensile strength of the membranous labyrinth (breakage pressure) in real cases. Table 3.3 shows the following threshold pressures: semicircular canal 1992.8 mmHg, utricular membrane 210.6 mmHg, Reissner's membrane 106.7–142.2 mmHg and saccular membrane 64.0 mmHg. According to these values, a certain elevation of endolymphatic pressure can cause hydrops only in the saccular and Reissner's membranes. Additionally, these data suggest that the pressure of endolymphatic space cannot be greater than the breakage pressure of the saccular membrane. In Table 3.4, blood pressure is shown in various blood vessels of the human vascular system for comparison [8]. Since the range of blood pressure is assumed to be the upper limit of physiological changes in the inner ear, the utricule and semicircular canals never break in a purely mechanical sense. In an extreme case, rupture could occur particularly in the saccular membrane. Endolymphatic pressure cannot be elevated over breakage pressure of the saccular

Table 3.3. Pressure at which breakage occurs in the human membranous labyrinth

Parts of labyrinth	Pressure (mmHg)
Semicircular canal	1992.8
Utricular membrane	210.6
Reissner's membrane	106.7–142.2
Saccular membrane	64.0

Table 3.4. Human blood pressure. From Guyton [8]

Vessels	Blood pressure (mmHg)
Aorta	80–120
Artery	80–120
Arteriole	40– 85
Capillary	(15)– 30
Venule	(10)– 15
Vein	(5)– 10
Vena cava	0 – 5

Numbers in *parentheses* are approximations.

membrane (64.0 mmHg); therefore, hydrops or rupture is easily developed at a pressure equivalent to that of the arteriolae.

Evidence on Mechanical Properties of Labyrinth in Temporal Bone Pathology

We now describe 2 cases [9, 10], suggesting that the saccular membrane is the weakest and that the endolymphatic pressure cannot exceed the breakage pressure of the saccule.

Case 1

A 38-year-old male died of a leukemoid reaction due to bone metastasis of gastric cancer [9]. A few weeks before death, the platelet number became extremely low. He suddenly developed total deafness in the left ear 13 days prior to death. The next day hearing in the right ear was completely absent. He became totally deaf and did not recover from deafness before his death.

Histopathological Findings in the Right Temporal Bone. A massive bleeding was observed both in the perilymphatic and endolymphatic spaces (Fig. 3.6). Reissner's membrane was distended by blood in the chochlear duct, but no rupture of Reissner's membrane was detected (Fig. 3.6). Although the tunnel and supporting elements were preserved in the organ of Corti, outer hair cells were missing. The tectorial membrane disappeared in most turns, but was found to be elevated and deviated. Bleeding was observed in the spiral ligament of the basal and middle turns. The stria vascularis in the basal turn was filled with blood and marginal cell lining was disrupted where the blood had spouted into the cochlear duct. The modiolus and spiral ligament were filled with blood which had leaked into the perilymphatic space. The saccule and the perilymphatic spaces in the vestibule were occupied by blood. The blood had gushed into the lumen from the subepithelial tissue of the saccule and the otolith and otolith membrane were dislocated into the blood mass. The saccular membrane was ruptured(Fig. 3.7). The endolymphatic hemorrhage

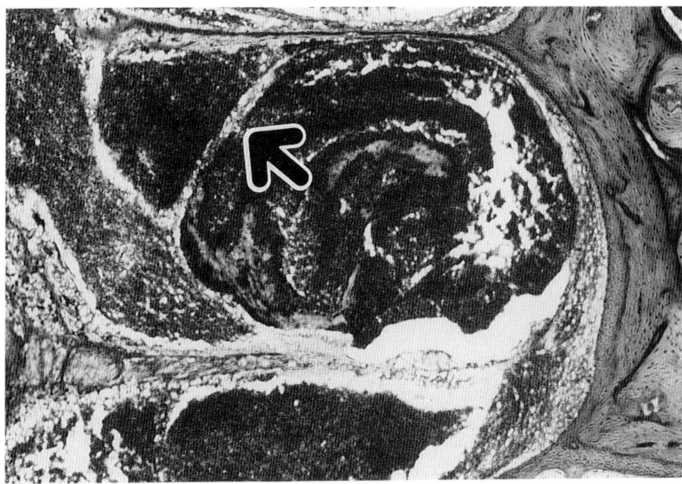

Fig. 3.6. Cochlea of the right temporal bone in case 1. The cochlear duct is filled with blood. Reissner's membrane (*arrow*) is distended, but did not rupture

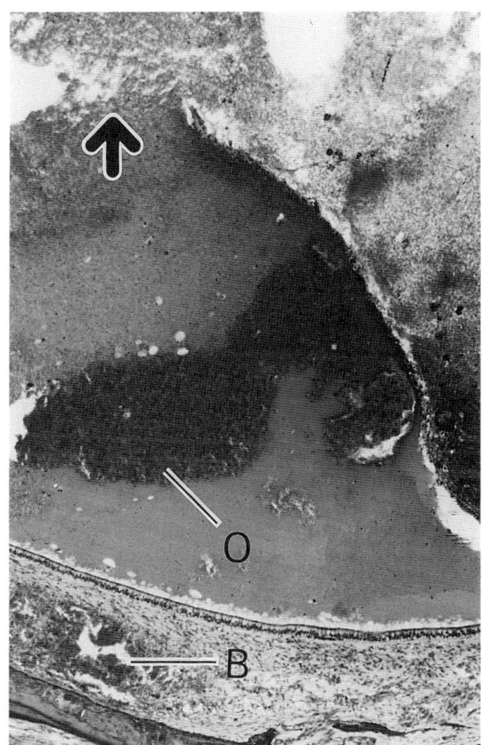

Fig. 3.7. Saccule of the right ear in case 1. Blood and exudate fill the lumen and the membrane is broken (*arrow*). *O*, otolith and otolith membrane; *B*, site of bleeding

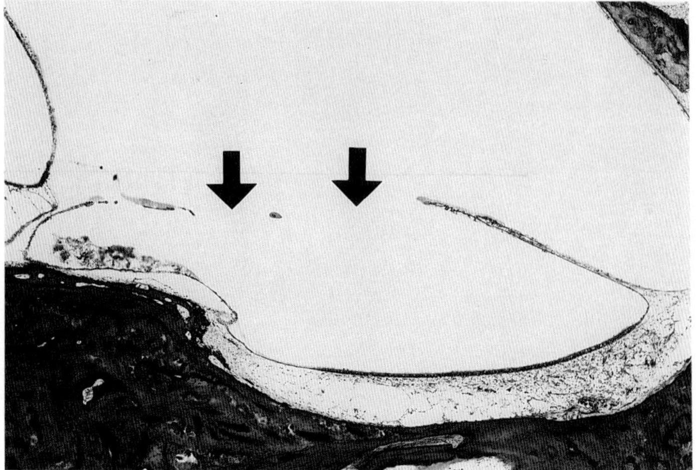

Fig. 3.8. Large defect of the saccular membrane (*arrows*) in the left ear of case 2

in this ear apparently resulted from a rupture of the small blood vessels of the stria vascularis and the subepithelial tissue of the saccule (Fig. 3.7). In consideration of the fact that Reissner's membrane did not break, the bleeding must have occurred in the arteriole.

Case 2

A 52-year-old male died of a metastatic cancer of the stomach [10]. One year before death, he developed vertigo of sudden onset. He had to rest for 3 days because of nausea and anorexia. Otological examinations were not performed.

Histopathological Findings in the Left Temporal Bone. Pathological findings were observed in the membranous labyrinth of this ear. A large portion of the saccular membrane was found to have disappeared (Fig. 3.8). A microscopic observation of the ruptured margins showed that this defect of the membrane was not an artifact. The otolith and otolith membrane were lost, while their fragmented tissues were present within the saccule near the saccular duct (Fig. 3.8). The macula sacculi became thin and sensory cells and nerve fibers decreased in number. In the cochlea, Reissner's membrane was extended and partially depressed, but it was not ruptured (Fig. 3.9). The saccular wall was ruptured. These findings suggest that endolymphatic hydrops of the pars inferior was present previous to a big volume loss.

Summary

The mechanical properties of the human membranous labyrinth were evaluated by a microtension measuring device developed in our laboratory. Since the saccular

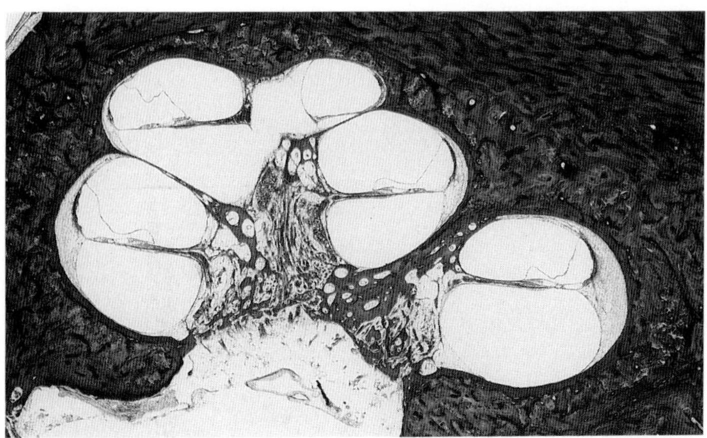

Fig. 3.9. The left cochlea of case 2 shows distension and partial collapse of Reissner's membrane. There is no visible rupture

and Reissner's membranes are the weakest sites mechanically, a certain elevation of the endolymphatic pressure of labyrinth can cause hydrops only in the pars inferior. Also, the pressure of the endolymphatic space cannot exceed 64.0 mmHg, which is the upper limit of the breakage pressure of the saccule. Temporal bone examinations of 2 cases were described, showing that the saccular membrane was ruptured, and the Reissner's membrane was extended but intact.

References

1. Hallpike CS, Cairns H (1938) Observations on the pathology of Ménière's syndrome. J Laryngol Otol 53:625–655
2. Gussen R (1973) Pathology of Ménière's disease: Further studies. Ann Otol Rhinol Laryngol 82:179–181
3. Altmann F, Kornfeld M (1965) Histological studies of Ménière's disease. Ann Otol Rhinol Laryngol 74:915–943
4. Schuknecht HF, Benitez JT, Beekhuis J (1962) Further observations on the pathology on Ménière's disease. Ann Otol Rhinol Laryngol 71:1039–1053
5. Tonndorf J (1976) Endolymphatic hydrops. Mechanical causes of hearing loss. Arch Otorhinolaryngol 212:293–299
6. Yamamoto N, Ishii T, Machida T (1990) Measurement of the mechanical properties of the tympanic membranes with a microtension tester. Acta Otolaryngol 110:85–91
7. Yamamoto N, Ishii T, Machida T (to be published) Mechanical properties of membranous labyrinth.
8. Guyton AC (1986) Texbook of medical physiology. Saunders, Philadelphia, pp 218–220
9. Ishii T, Toriyama M, Takiguchi T (1983) Pathological findings in the cochlear duct due to endolymphatic hemorrhage. Adv Otorhinolaryngol 31:148–154
10. Igarashi Y, Ishii T (1982) Histopathology of Ménière's disease with rupture of saccular membrane (in Japanese). Pract Otol (Kyoto) 75 (Suppl 3):1218–1225

Chapter 4

Blood-Flow Regulation in the Vestibulum and Inner Ear Microvasculature in Experimental Hydrops: A Scanning Electron Microscopic Study

Yoshiaki Nakai, Haruhiko Masutani, Masahiko Sugita, Makoto Moriguchi, and Kazuhiro Matsunaga

Blood-flow regulation in the inner ear, particularly the cochlea, has been the subject of many studies reported so far, and the special characteristics of capillary plexuses and arteriovenous (AV) anastomoses in the stria vascularis and spiral ligament are well known. With regard to the vestibule, on the other hand, basic studies on blood flow regulation have been insufficient and incomplete, although reports are available on unique features of blood vessels. In some cases of dizziness due to vestibular disorder, circulatory disturbance of the vestibule has been implicated as the underlying cause and, in fact, circulatory agents are in common use in the treatment of the condition.

As is obvious from reading the above, it seems of great importance, both fundamentally and clinically, to investigate blood-flow regulation in the vestibule. The present study investigates blood-flow regulation in the inner ear, particularly the vestibule, from the morphological viewpoint by using the casting method. In a further attempt to study local blood-flow impairment or local vascular disturbance in the inner ear occurring in association with inner ear disorder, experimental endolymphatic hydrops was produced in animals, and the microvasculature of the inner ear was observed using the casting method.

Materials and Methods

Twenty Hartley guinea pigs weighing 250–300 g were used. Upon thoracostomy of the animals under general anesthesia, a cannula was inserted into the left ventricle, through which 30 ml of Mercox resin was injected. After the resin hardened, the temporal bone was removed, deprived of tissue surrounding the cast by dissolution in 6*N*-hydrochloric acid, processed in the usual manner (drying and Au-coating), and observed with a scanning electron microscope (SEM). Some of the temporal bones were embedded in stylene resin and subsequently cut into sections. The rest of the blocks, after having been cleared of stylene resin with propylene oxide, were prepared in the usual manner and examined by SEM.

In addition, we induced experimental hydrops (right side) in 5 guinea pigs by cauterizing the endolymphatic sac with 10% silver nitrate (Yazawa et al.'s method [1]) and observed their inner ear vessels by SEM using the casting method. In the present study, the animals were used at 2 months after the experimental production of the hydrops, their left inner ears serving as controls.

Results

The wall of the vestibular artery was thick and consisted of several layers, and there was little perivascular space. The inner surface of the artery was elevated by clearly demarcated endothelial cells and their nuclei (Fig. 4.1). The veins of the vestibule, on the other hand, were exceedingly thin walled, and there was an ample space between the veins and surrounding bony walls wherein abundant reticular connective tissue was noted (Fig. 4.2). Immediately before the neuroepithelial area the arterioles formed complex coils. These vessels resembled coiled arterioles of the cochlea (Fig. 4.3). On the basement membrane side of the capillary plexus immediately subjacent to the epithelium of the utricular macula, arterioles stemming from the anterior vestibular artery were noted to run almost straight and to communicate with the venous system without branching or forming anastomoses. These various vessels, because of their morphological characteristics, were considered to be AV anastomoses (Fig. 4.4). In the saccular macula, on the other hand, no distinct AV anastomoses existed on the basement membrane side while two-layered capillary networks were formed on the cochlear side (Fig. 4.5). In the semicircular ampullae, especially at the junction of the lateral and anterior ampullae, several arterioles that represent a terminal portion of the anterior vestibular

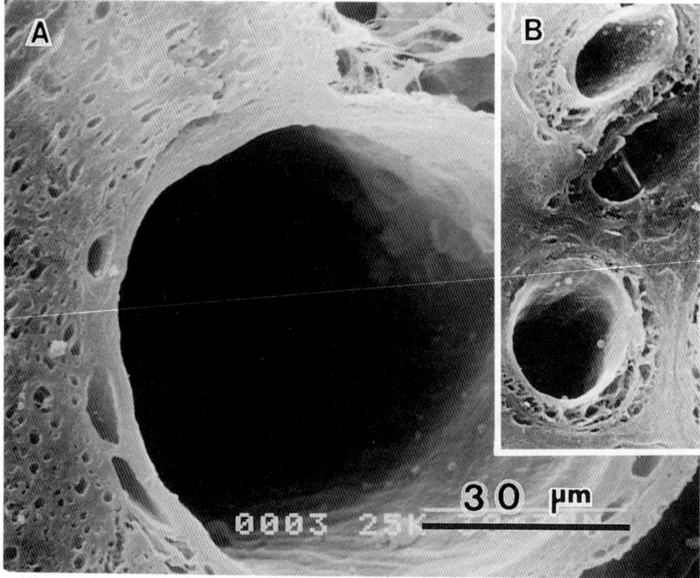

Fig. 4.1A, B. The vascular walls of the **A** anterior vestibular artery and **B** arterioles are thick and little perivascular space is observed

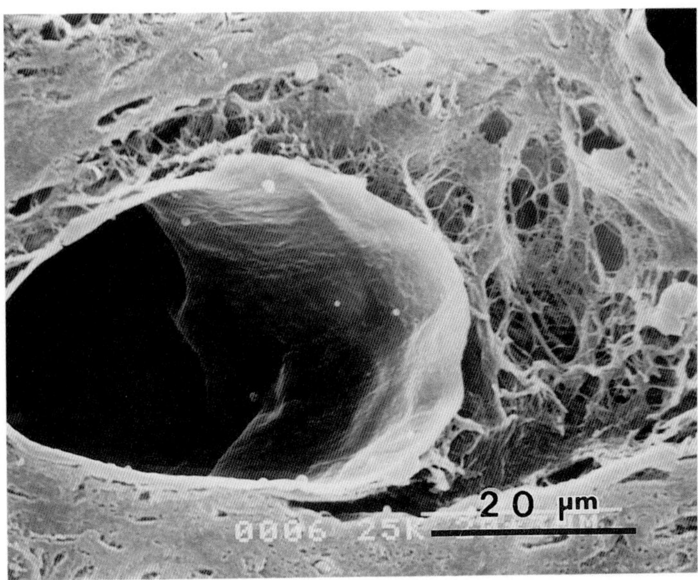

Fig. 4.2. Vestibular vein. The vascular wall of the vein is very thin. The perivascular space, which contains abundant reticular connective tissue, is wide

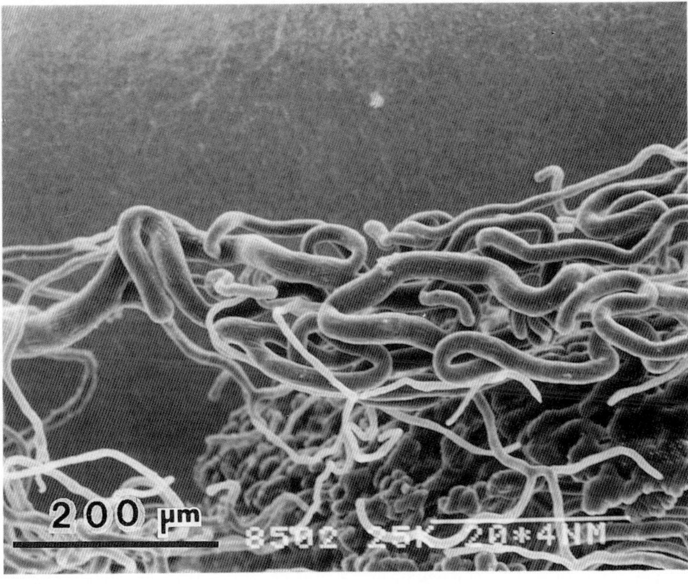

Fig. 4.3. Coiled arterioles in the vestibule. Immediately before the neuroepithelial area the arterioles form complex coils

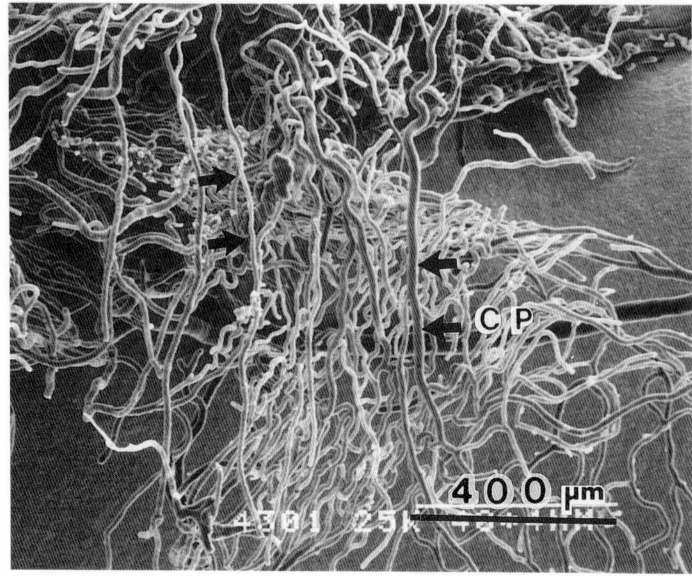

Fig. 4.4. Microvasculature in the utricle. Arteriovenous anastomosis (*arrows*) is observed below the capillary plexus (*CP*)

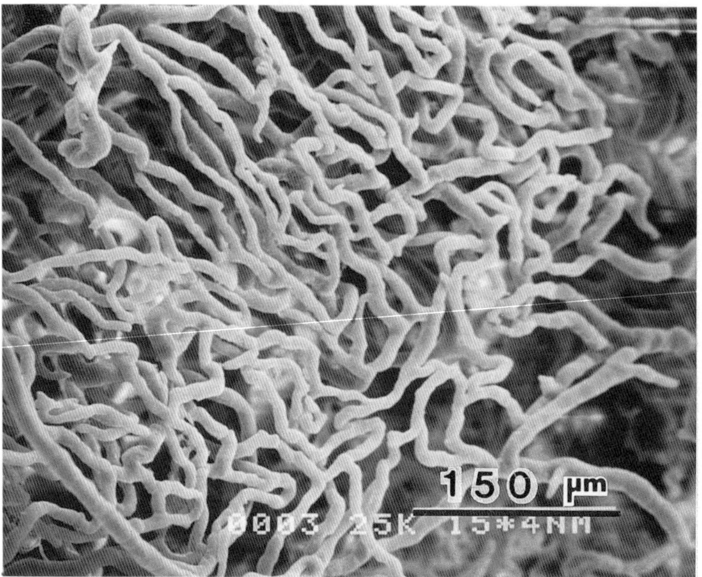

Fig. 4.5. Microvasculature in the saccule. A dense capillary plexus is observed, but no arteriovenous anastomosis exist

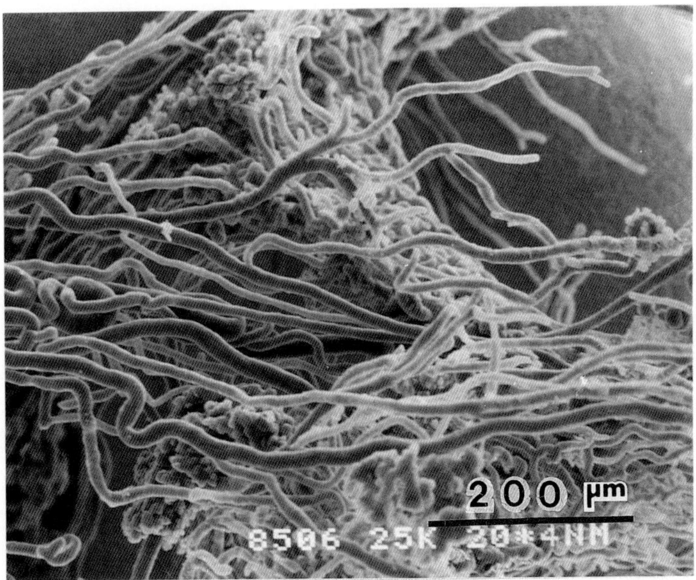

Fig. 4.6. Microvasculature near the superior and lateral semicircular ampulla. Nearly linear vessels without anastomosis are observed

artery were seen running in almost straightlines without forming connections with the microvasculature of the ampullae (Fig. 4.6).

At 2 months after the production of experimental endolymphatic hydrops, the vascular structure on the lateral cochlear walls was noted to have undergone changes that varied from place to place even in the same turn of the same animal. Thus, within the same turn, the dilatation of capillaries of the stria vascularis and the narrowing of vessels at AV anastomoses of the spiral ligament were prominent when compared to the control side in some places, while, conversely, the narrowing of capillaries of the vascular stria and the dilatation of vessels at AV anastomoses of the spiral ligament were evident in others. Moreover, there were areas where no marked changes in the vascular system were discernible (Fig. 4.7). In the saccular macula, notably on its epithelial side, vessels of the capillary plexus were found to be of reduced caliber. These changes were particularly pronounced at the center of the macula (Fig. 4.8). No vascular abnormalities in capillary plexuses and AV anastomoses as seen in the cochlea were observed in the utricular macula, nor were noteworthy abnormalities seen in capillaries of the semicircular ampullae or in vessels of the semicircular canal.

Discussion

Few reports are available to date concerning blood-flow regulation in the vestibule. Notwithstanding this lack, a correct understanding of the anatomic basis for

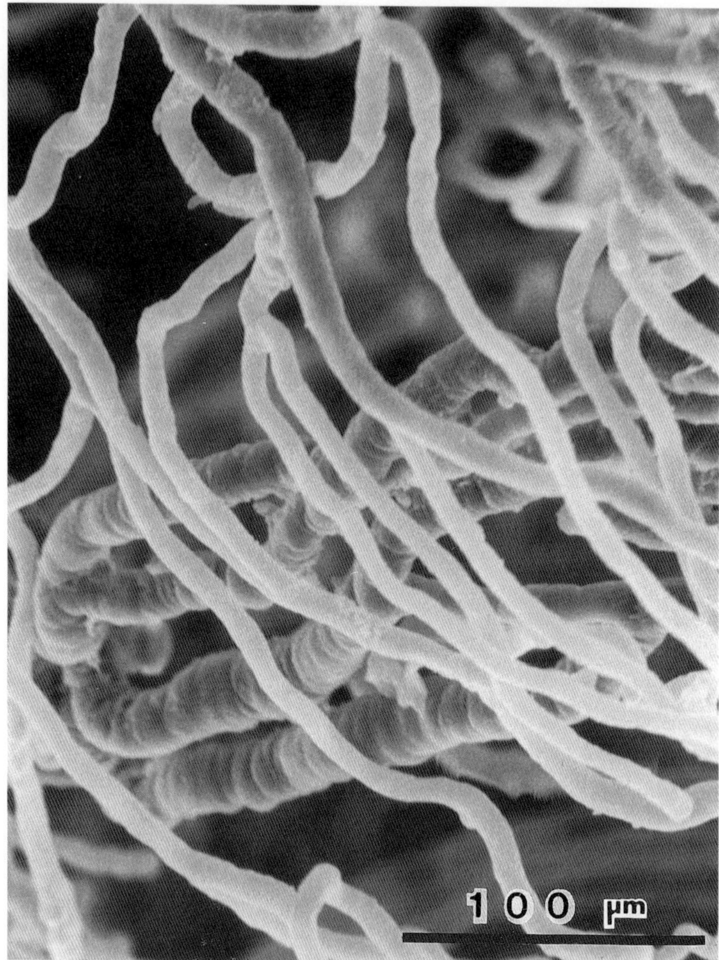

Fig. 4.7. Microvasculature of the lateral cochlear wall at 2 months after induction of experimental endolymphatic hydrops. Dilatation of capillaries on the stria vascularis and narrowing of vessels at the arteriovenous anastomosis of the spiral ligament are observed

blood-flow regulation not only in the cochlea but also in neuroepithelial areas of the vestibule is of great importance from both the fundamental and clinical viewpoints. In the vestibule, like in the cochlea, there is a characteristic blood vessel pattern over the entire length of the structure [2–4]. The coiling of arterioles in the vestibule, as in the upper and lower coiled arterioles of the cochlea, provides a blood pressure buffering function and, by virtue of its elongated blood vessels, favors the retention of blood, thereby ensuring constant blood supply to the neuroepithelial areas situated peripheral to the arterioles [5, 6].

The SEM findings of blood vessels of the vestibule by the stylene cracking method are interpreted as indicating that the vascular structure confers resilient blood-

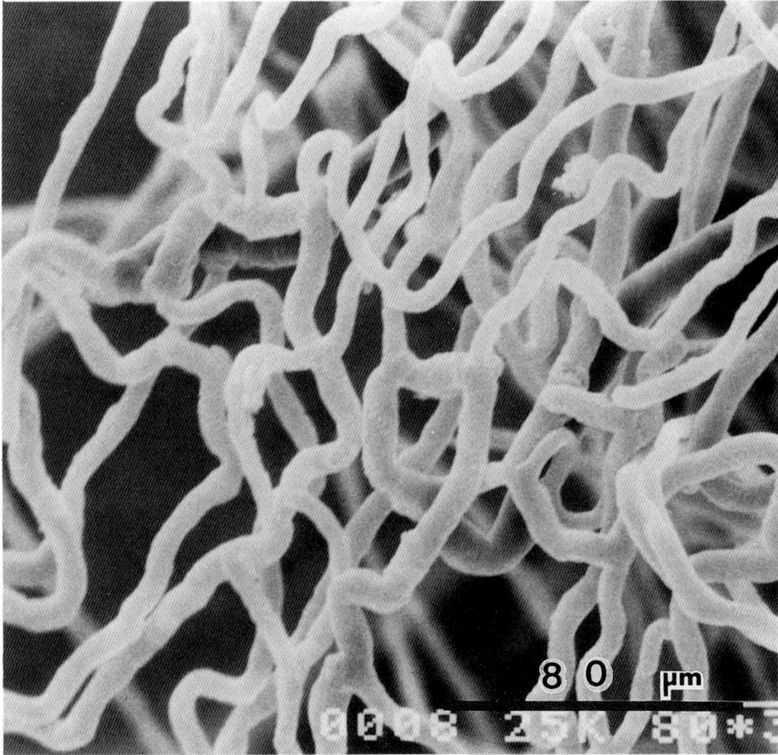

Fig. 4.8. Microvasculature in the saccular macula at 2 months after induction of experimental endolymphatic hydrops. On the epitherial side, the capillaries are found to be of reduced caliber

pumping function on the arterial system and sufficient distensibility on the venous system, thus serving the purpose of pooling blood.

Worthy of particular note among the present observations is the existence of AV anastomoses immediately subjacent to the capillary plexus of the utricular macula. These communicating vessels, like the capillary plexus and AV anastomoses of the stria vascularis and spiral ligament, are considered to subserve regulating blood flow to functional vessels, i.e., the capillary plexus. It thus became obvious that a regulatory mechanism of local blood flow really exists in the utricle, too (Fig. 4.9). A similar vascular structure that is affiliated with such functional vessels and serves as collateral pathways, so to speak, was noted to exist also at the junction of the ampullae of the anterior and lateral semicircular canals (Fig. 4.10).

In inner ears affected by endolymphatic hydrops, on the other hand, capillaries of the vascular stria and vessels of AV anastomoses of the spiral ligament were found to be of irregular caliber, and vessels of the capillary plexus of the sacular macula were narrowed. These findings point to the possibility that endolymphatic hydrops gives rise to circulatory disturbances of the lateral walls of the cochlea and

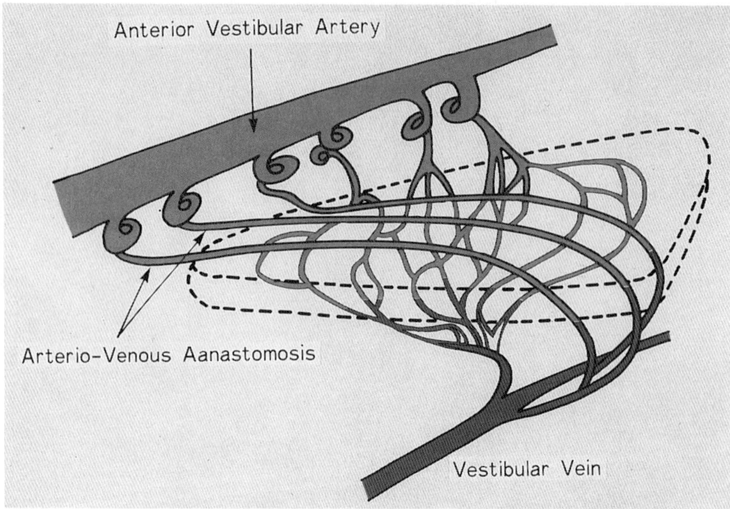

Fig. 4.9. Schema of the utricular vasculature

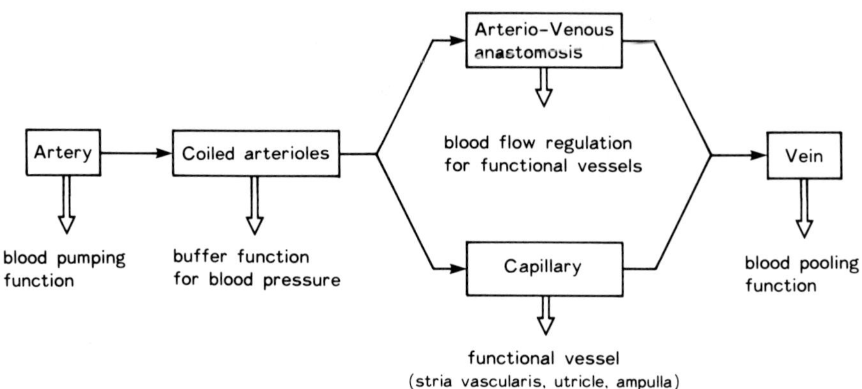

Fig. 4.10. Participation of the inner ear vessels in blood-flow regulation

of the saccular macula. Implicated as the cause of this circulatory impairment of the cochlea is damage to the vascular system on the outer wall of the cochlear duct at the attachment of Reissner's membrane. The damage arises from elevated endolymphatic pressure and stretching of the membrane [7].

The results of our present experimental study provide ample presumptive, although not definitive, evidence of circulatory disturbance occurring in the cochlear vascular system. In also seems possible, however, to interpret the vascular changes in the outer wall of the cochlear duct as a consequence of the operation of a local defense mechanism against a load of endolymphatic hydrops. The importance of AV anastomoses at the spiral ligament in the maintenance of blood supply to the stria vascularis is thus suggested.

In the vestibule, abnormalities in vascular structure were observed only in the saccular maculae. A possible anatomical explanation for this could be that while the utricular macula is partly separated from the bony labyrinth and is proportionately less liable to be subject to endolymphatic pressure, the saccular macula is in direct contact with the bony labyrinth and, accordingly, would be directly influenced by a rise in endolymphatic pressure. Furthermore, as mentioned earlier, AV anastomoses in the utricular macula, by virtue of their structural speciality, are capable of regulating blood flow and thereby serving as buffers preventing circulatory disturbance.

Summary

The microvasculature of the inner ear, especially the vestibule, was observed with a scanning electron microscope using the casting and stylene cracking methods. Alterations in the inner ear vasculature occurring in association with endolymphatic hydrops were also investigated. The results thus obtained are briefly summarized as follows:

1. In the vestibule, the arteries, coiled arterioles, and the veins are endowed with their respective characteristic morphologic features and play a role in the regulatory mechanisms of circulation as do those of the cochlea.
2. Arteriovenous anastomoses were demonstrated to exist in the utricular macula, a finding suggesting the existence of a regulatory mechanism of local blood flow.
3. Endolymphatic hydrops was noted to be associated preferentially with vascular abnormalities on the lateral wall of the cochlear duct and in the saccular macula, among other vestibular structures.

References

1. Yazawa Y, Shea J, Kitahera M (1985) Endolymphatic hydrops after cauterizing the sac with silver nitrate. Arch Otolaryngol 111:301–304
2. Smith CA (1953) The capillaries of the vestibular membranous labyrinth in the guinea pig. Laryngoscope 63:87–104
3. Nakai Y, Masutani H, Ohashi K (1983) Observation of the microvascular structure of the vestibular organ by scanning electron microscope (in Japanese). Pract Otol (Kyoto) 76:2248–2263
4. Masutani H, Ohashi K, Nakai Y (1984) The observation of the microvascular structure of the vesibular organ (in Japanese). Ear Res Jpn 15:116–118
5. Masutani H (1986) Microvascular structure of the inner ear (in Japanese). Ear Res Jpn 17:8–12
6. Nakai Y, Masutani H, Cho H (1986) Scanning electron microscopy of the microvascular system in the inner ear. Scan Electron Microsc 2:543–548
7. Matsunaga K, Masutani H, Nakai Y (1989) Observation of inner ear vessels in experimental hydrops (in Japanese). Equilibrium Res [Suppl] 5:112–115

CHAPTER 5

Electrophysiological Aspects of Surgically-Induced Endolymphatic Hydrops

Jun Kusakari, Zenya Ito, Norihide Nishikawa, Minoru Takeyama, Yasuo Furuhashi, Akira Hara, Tetsuaki Kawase, Kenji Ohyama, Toshimitsu Kobayashi, Eiichi Arakawa, and Masaaki Rokugo

Endolymphatic hydrops, a characteristic finding in Ménière's disease can be induced in guinea pigs by surgical obliteration of the endolymphatic duct and sac. Since the reports by Harada [1], Naito [2], and Kimura [3], this hydropic animal has frequently been used as an animal model of Ménière's disease. The purpose of the present paper is to summarize the results of our 10-year study on these animals [4–9] and to review the recently published articles by other investigators. In the present study, endolymphatic hydrops was induced in 136 albino guinea pigs by obliterating the endolymphatic duct and sac. The presence of the hydrops was histologically confirmed in a majority of the cases (Fig. 5.1). The endolymphatic potential (EP) was recorded through the round window and the recording electrode for other cochlear potentials was placed at the round window. The sound stimuli were clicks generated by a 90 μs rectangular pulse and tone bursts of 0.5–16 kHz with a 1 ms rise-fall time and a 10 ms duration. Similar methods were used in the majority of the reports reviewed in the present paper. Therefore, the methods or the conditions of the experiments used elsewhere will be described only when they differ from ours.

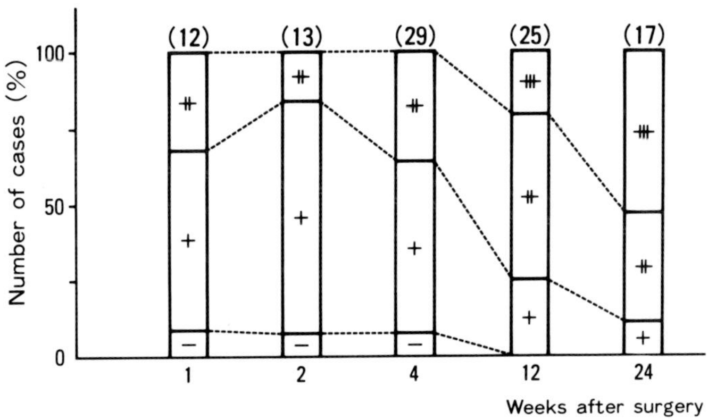

Fig. 5.1. The extent of hydrops in the basal turn as a function of the postoperative time. –, no hydrops; +, slights; + +, moderate; + + +, extensive; ( ), number of cases

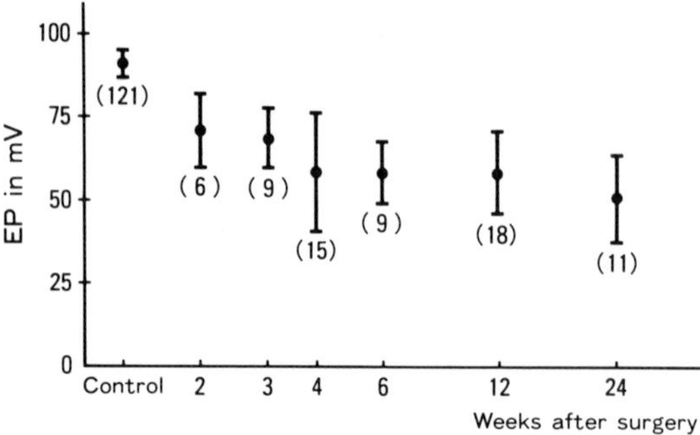

Fig. 5.2. The level of the endolymphatic potential (*EP*) (mean ±SD) as a function of the postoperative time. ( ), number of cases

Endolymphatic Potential

Figure 5.2 shows the postoperative time-related changes of the EP in hydropic ears. The *circles* and *vertical bars* indicate the means and standard deviations (SD) of our data, respectively. These findings are in close agreement with the results reported by other investigators [10–13]. Namely, a significant reduction of the EP was already seen at the end of the 2nd postoperative week. The potential further declined thereafter and reached a plateau in animals at 4 weeks. The level of the EP in animals at 24 weeks was 50.7 ± 13.1 mV. Most investigators believe that the EP is the sum of two potentials of opposite polarity, i.e., a positive electrogenic K^+ secretion potential (+KSP) (+120 to +130 mV) and a negative K^+ diffusion potential (−KDP) (−30 to −40 mV). Consequently, the reduction of the EP magnitude means the decrease of +KSP, the increase of −KDP, or both. Since +KSP is produced at the stria vascularis by an active transport mechanism, this potential is rapidly abolished by anoxia. When the hydropic ear was subjected to asphyxia, the EP decreased slower than in the normal control, and the decline rate of the potential was approximately proportional to the level of the EP [5]. The correlation coefficient between the reduced amount of the EP after 2-min asphyxia and the level of the EP before asphyxia was 0.760 (n = 30) (Fig. 5.3a, b). A similar phenomenon was also observed in ethacrynic acid-intoxicated animals [14]. These results indicate that the energy utilization is inhibited at the stria vascularis. Another phenomenon suggesting the strial dysfunction is the increased susceptibility of the EP to furosemide in hydropic ears. The maximally reduced amount of the EP from the preadministration level by 50 mg/kg furosemide was significantly larger in hydropic ears than in normal controls ($P < 0.05$) (Fig. 5.4). Furthermore, the recovery of the EP after reaching the maximally reduced level was delayed in hydropic ears when 80 mg/kg furosemide was given. Although there were no significant differences between the 3-to 12-week-postoperative animals and the normal controls, the maximum rate of the EP recovery was significantly slower in the 24-week-postoperative animals than in the normal controls (2.8 ± 1.2 mV/min versus 8.2 ± 1.9 mV/min; $P < 0.01$) [9]. Recent morphological studies on hydropic

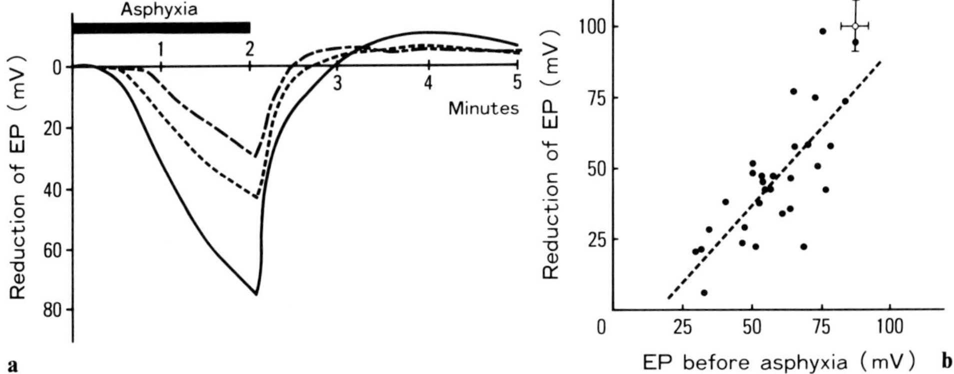

Fig. 5.3. a The response of the endolymphatic potential (*EP*) to 2 – min asphyxia in hydropic ears in guinea pigs 2 (———), 4 (----), and 12 (—–—) weeks postoperatively **b** The reduced amount of the EP after 2 – min asphyxia as a function of the preasphyxic level of the endolymphatic potential (*EP*). $r = 0.76$; $y = 1.1x - 18.0$; o, values in normal control ($n = 10$)

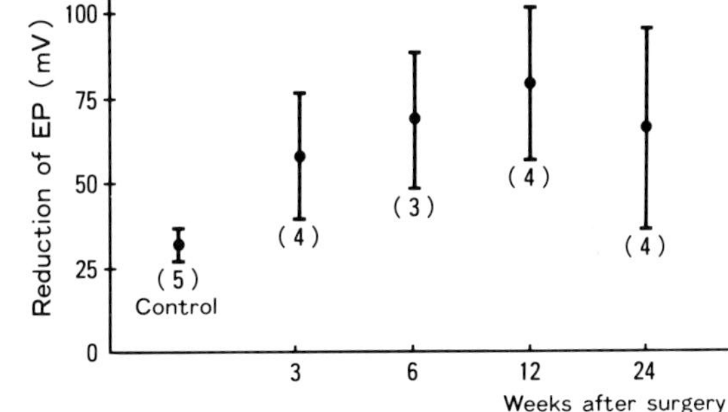

Fig. 5.4. Maximally reduced amount of the endolymphatic potential (*EP*) from the preadministration value by 50 mg/kg furosemide (mean ±SD). ( ), number of cases

ears have also demonstrated the postoperative time-related changes in the stria vascularis [15]. Based on the above reasons, it is highly likely that the strial dysfunction is a major factor in reducing the EP.

– KDP is determined by the ionic composition of the cochlear fluid and the ionic permeability in the endolymph-perilymph barrier. Although there are some reports indicating the increase of Na^+ in the endolymph of hydropic ears, most authors agree that the ionic composition in the endolymph (Na^+ and K^+) remains unchanged in hydropic ears [10, 11].

Information on the permeability of the membrane is rather limited. The endolymphatic potential of the saccule (SEP) is only 5 mV in magnitude, and its anoxia-sensitive positive part is attributed to the potential leakage from the cochlea. In normal animals, the potential is reduced to one-tenth of its original value when it reaches the saccule. When the animal was subjected to anoxia or given loop diuretics, the response pattern in the SEP was quite similar to that of the EP

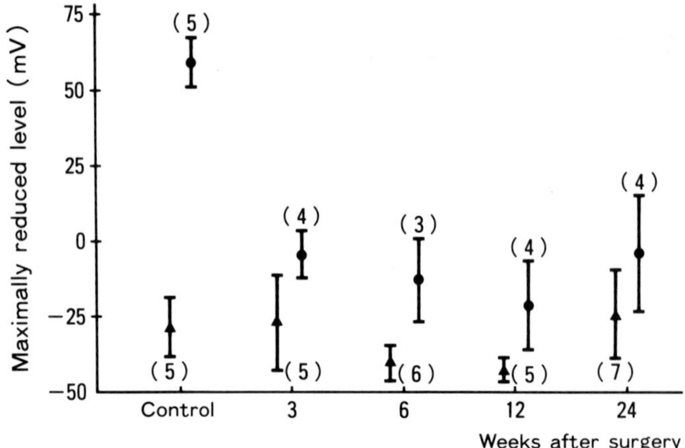

Fig. 5.5. Maximally reduced level of the endolymphatic potential by furosemide (mean ±SD). ●, 50 mg/kg; ▲, 80 mg/kg

although the absolute value of the potential change in the former was almost one-tenth that of the latter[5, 16]. Similar findings were observed in an earlier stage of hydrops (2–4 weeks postoperatively), whereas a different SEP response pattern from that of the EP was seen in later stages (4–12 weeks). These results indicate that the membrane of the ductus reuniens becomes more penetrable to the electric current due to the increased ionic permeability, and that the transmission of the EP to the saccule is supressed in advanced hydrops. However, the studies on other parts of the endolymph-perilymph barrier show no alternation in the ionic permeability of hydropic ears. Konishi, Salt, and Kimura [11] have reported no change in the permeability and conductance of K^+ ion between the scala media and the scala tympani of the hydropic ears. Another method to examine the change in −KDP is to determine the level of the EP when +KSP is totally abolished by anoxia or loop diuretics. Figure 5.5 shows the maximally reduced level of the EP by furosemide in the hydropic ears with various postoperative periods. The EP was reduced to −30 to −40 mV by 80 mg/kg of furosemide in the hydropic ears as well as in the normal controls [9]. A 4-week-postoperative animal in our series exhibited a reduction of the EP to −43 mV within 20 min after the onset of anoxia. Konishi, Salt, and Kimura [11] have also reported that the maximally reduced level of the EP by anoxia in the hydropic ears was at almost the same level as that in the sham-operated ears. Taking these results into consideration, it is highly likely that −KDP is not changed in hydropic ears and the reduction of the EP is solely due to the supression of +KSP, i.e., strial dysfunction.

In contrast to the consistent values of Na^+ and K^+, the Ca^{2+} concentration in the endolymph is significantly elevated in hydropic ears according to Ninoyu and Meyer zum Gottesberge [17]. They measured the endolymphatic Ca^{2+} activity at the 3rd turn of the cochlea with hydrops 12–15 months postoperatively and clearly demonstrated a significant elevation of Ca^{2+} in hydropic ears (1.01×10^{-4} *M*) in comparison with the normal value (2.6×10^{-5} *M*). Furthermore, there was a striking correlation between the elevation of Ca^{2+} and the reduction of the EP or the increase in volume in the scala media. However, it is yet to be determined whether this increase of Ca^{2+} in the endolymph is directly coupled to the suppression of the EP, because only a slight reduction of the EP has been reported in the animals exposed to an intense sound in which the Ca^{2+} activity in the endolymph is increased to the level of $0.5–1.0 \times 10^{-3}$ *M* [18].

Cochlear Microphonics

The reports on the cochlear microphonics (CM) are limited in contrast to the large number of studies on the other cochlear potentials of hydropic ears. Klis and Smoorenburg [19] have reported that the CM amplitude of the maximum response is reduced but the threshold remains within normal limits in animals 4 months postoperatively. Similar cases were reported by Horner and Cazals [20]. On the contrary, several authors have reported that the input-output curves are totally suppressed progressively with the time elapsed after the surgery, at low frequency (500 Hz) as well as at high frequencies (4–8 kHz) [21–23]. Our results support the latter findings. Although the threshold shift was smaller in the CM than in the compound action potential (AP), the changes in both potentials were well correlated at all frequencies [6]. Recent morphological studies clearly demonstrated the damage in outer hair cells of hydropic ears [24]. It is highly likely that the main cause of the CM suppression is the damage of the outer hair cells per se in addition to the reduction of the EP.

Compound Action Potential

Progressive hearing loss is one characteristic symptom of Ménière's disease. The compound action potential (AP) threshold, which is considered to reflect the hearing of hydropic animals, has been reported by many investigators. Uno [21] described a progressive suppression of the AP amplitude with postoperative time. Kumagami and Miyazaki [23] described the elevation of the threshold after 4 weeks and Morizono, Cohen, and Sikora [25] also reported a significant difference in threshold between animals of more than 60 days and those of less than 60 days postoperative time. van Deelen et al. [26] found no change in the AP of animals at 1 month but a 10–20 dB elevation in animals at 2 months and a 10–40 dB elevation in animals at 4–8 months. Horner and Cazals [27] have clearly demonstrated the progressive elevation of the threshold using long-term implanted electrodes. Figure 5.6 shows the threshold of the click-evoked AP (peak equivalent sound pressure level to evoke the amplitude of 10 μV) in our animals at various postoperative times. Although the values varied considerably among individual animals, the mean threshold shift increased progressively with time after surgery. These results are similar to those reported by other authors.

As for the relation of the threshold shift to the morphological changes, our results exhibited the close correlation between the threshold shift and the extent of hydrops

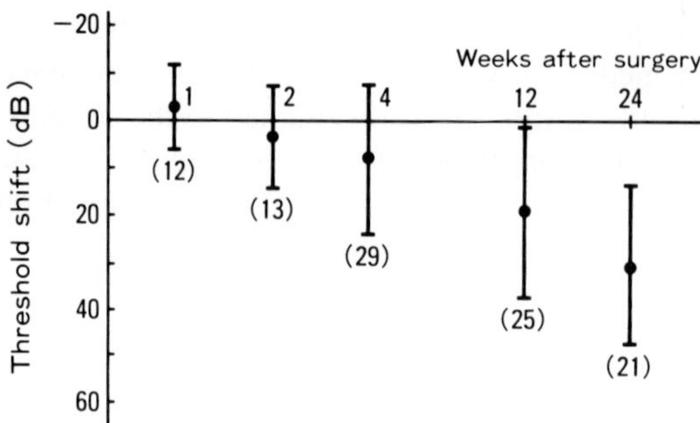

Fig. 5.6. Mean and SD of the threshold shift from the normal value in the click-evoked action potential (AP). ( ), number of cases

[4, 6]. Similar findings were reported by Takeda [28] and Morizono et al. [25]. However, the experiments using rabbits [29] and rats [30] have shown that the threshold shift exhibits no apparent correlation with the extent of hydrops but rather closely correlates with the atrophy of sensory hair cells and/or spiral ganglions. Aran et al. [31] have described contradictory results. They demonstrated a case which exhibited (59 days postoperatively) the elevated threshold at all frequencies ranging from 0.5–32 kHz with a significant loss of hair cells only at the apex. Still controversial is the generating mechanism of the AP threshold elevation in the hydopic ears. The reduction of the EP is one of the contributing factors. However, it is reasonable to think that other, more important factor(s) must be present if we consider the different time course of the suppression between the AP and the EP (Figs. 5.2, 5.6).

Low-tone hearing loss at the early stage is another characteristic symptom of Ménière's disease, and several investigators described the presence of low-tone deafness in the early stage of the hydrops. Morizono et al. [25] reported the elevation of the AP threshold only below 4 kHz in the animals within 60 postoperative days. Horner and Cazals [27] have found threshold elevations up to 20 dB for frequencies between 250 Hz–6.4 kHz within the 2nd postoperative week, whereas the threshold above 8 kHz remained unchanged. However, Martin et al. [29] have reported different results in auditory evoked brainstem response of rabbits, i.e., mild to profound losses in low and high frequencies with relatively little change in the threshold at 2–4 kHz. In experiments using guinea pigs, various patterns in the AP audiogram were reported by other authors [32]. Figure 5.7 shows the threshold shift at each frequency in the animals which exhibited a significant elevation in the threshold of the click-evoked AP. The threshold shift was larger at higher frequencies than at lower ones in the 6-month-postoperative animals as well as in those at 3 months or less. In our animals, there was no finding suggesting the presence of low-tone hearing loss in either group.

Fluctuation of hearing is also commonly seen in Ménière's disease in humans. Observation using long-term, implanted electrodes is suitable for detecting the presence or absence of fluctuation in the AP threshold. Aran et al. [31] have reported a case with the fluctuating AP threshold ranging over all of the frequencies. Horner and Cazals [27] have also reported the fluctuation limited to low-to mid-frequencies and added that the extent of the fluctuation amounts to as much as 25 dB over a period of 24 h.

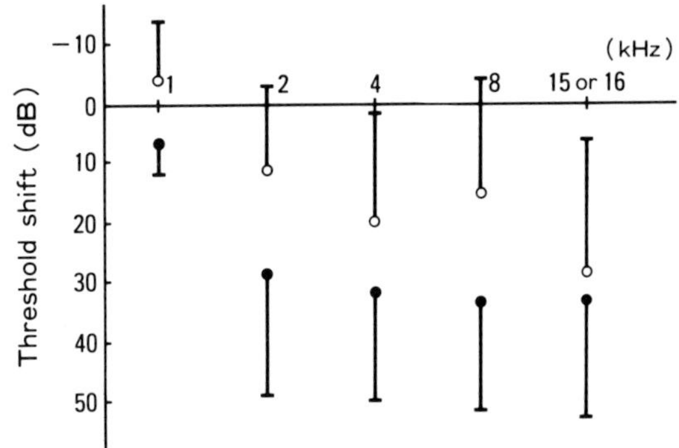

Fig. 5.7. Mean and SD of the threshold shift in the tone burst-evoked action potential (AP) in animals 6 months postoperatively (●; $n = 16$) and at 3 months or less (○; $n = 10$)

Many authors have reported the recruitment of the AP amplitude in the early stages, i.e., the threshold elevation, the steep growth values in the input-output curve, and the unchanged maximal amplitude [20, 26, 31]. These phenomena are reminiscent of recruitment in hearing in Ménière's disease in humans. It has also been reported that the AP amplitude decreases at all intensities in the advanced stages. Recruitment of the AP amplitude was observed in one-half of our cases in which the AP threshold was significantly elevated [4].

Summarizing these results, the surgically induced hydropic ear exhibits many audiological findings which are frequently observed in Ménière's disease in humans.

Summating Potential

Electrocochleograms of Ménière's disease frequently show the dominant negative summating potential (DNSP) which appears as a negative deflection before the AP wave-form. In normal guinea pigs, the polarity of a click-evoked summating potential (SP) is always positive when the potential is recorded at the round window. In our hydropic animals, the polarity of the click-evoked SP recorded at the round window was never negative in polarity, irrespective of the intensity of the click. Kumagami et al. [22] observed the negative SP in some animals with extensive hydrops, but the amplitude of the SP was so small that the wave-form of the SP-AP complex was quite different from that seen in human Ménière's disease. Reviewing the literature, it can be seen that many authors agree with the absence of a typical DNSP in surgically induced hydropic ears [26, 31, 33]. In contrast to these findings, the immunologically induced hydropic ears exhibit a different result. Ohashi et al. [34] succeeded in inducing the endolymphatic hydrops in 4 out of 11 animals by challenging the antigen to the ear of collagen II-sensitized animals and clearly demonstrated a DNSP in all cases. These results indicate that endolymphatic hydrops is not the single cause of the DNSP and that some other additional factors are necessary to elicit this characteristic potential.

When the potential was evoked by a tone burst with a high intensity, the polarities of the SP at the round window were negative at 500 Hz, negative or positive at 1 kHz, and positive above 2 kHz in the untreated animals. However, some hydropic animals in our experiment exhibited a positive SP at 500 kHz. This finding is most frequently observed in animals 1 week postoperatively (8 animals out of 9), and the incidence decreased thereafter [5]. This result may reflect the phenomenon relating to the pressure in the endolymphatic space. Further discussion on this phenomenon will be presented later (see "Effect of Intra-Cochlear Pressure").

Glycerol Effect

It is widely known that glycerol improves the hearing of patients with Ménière's disease at an early stage. However, the AP threshold of our hydropic animals (6 months after the surgery) was not improved but rather worsened by an i.v. administration of 3 g/kg glycerol [4, 8]. Although one case of improvement after glycerol was reported [32], Horner and Cazals [35] experienced results similar to ours. It is also known that advanced hearing loss in Ménière's disease is not improved by glycerol. Therefore, our negative results for the glycerol effect may relate to the fact that the experiment was performed in the animals long after the surgery. In contrast to the negative effect on the AP, the amplitude of the tone burst-evoked SP was markedly reduced [4]. Similar results were reported by several investigators [28, 35]. As previously mentioned, shortly after the surgery some animals showed the positive polarity in the SP evoked by a 500 Hz tone burst [6]. The glycerol effect upon such SP was examined in 11 animals, but the polarity was not reversed, with the exception of 1 animal.

Effect of Intra-Cochlear Pressure

Figure 5.8 shows the effect of intra-cochlear pressure upon the 500 Hz CM threshold recorded at the third turn of normal controls and hydropic ears. The hydrostatic pressure of 300 mm H_2O was exerted to the cochlea via a glass pipette at the scala tympani of the basal turn. The threshold elevation of about 20 dB was induced by the pressure in normal controls, while only a minimal shift (1.6 ± 2.6 dB) was observed in animals 4–6 days after surgery. This effect of hydrops decreased thereafter and the normal value was reattained in animals 3 months after surgery.

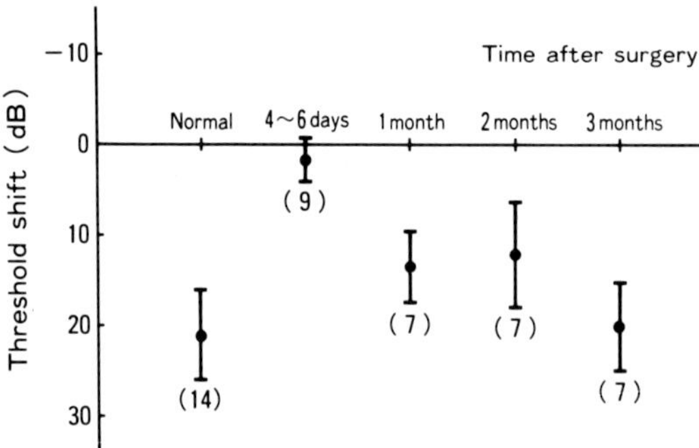

Fig. 5.8. Threshold shift at 500 Hz cochlear microphonics (CM) by a pressure application (300 mm H_2O) to the scala tympani. ( ), number of cases

Similar results were obtained in the Gellé tests of patients with Ménière's disease. When the pressure of 400 mm H_2O was applied to the external auditory canal, the bone conduction threshold of 500 Hz was elevated by about 10 dB in normal subjects. However, this effect was not observed in Ménière's disease cases when the hearing was reduced at the low frequencies [7]. Long and Morizono [36] described a small but definite increase in the intra-cochlear pressure in the early stage of hydrops (less than 6 days) and no significant change at the later stages. This absence of pressure effect upon the 500 Hz CM and the positive polarity of the 500 Hz SP in the early stage of hydrops may be a phenomenon reflecting the increased intra-cochlear pressure secondary to hydrops.

Effect of Acoustic Trauma

The effect of an intense sound (2 kHz, 110–120 dB, 30 min) upon the AP threshold was examined at frequencies ranging from 2–16 kHz in both the untreated ears and the hydropic ones in the 6th postoperative month. The hydropic ears, compared with the untreated ears, exhibited two different reactions to acoustic overstimulation (Fig. 5.9). First, the hydopic ears were less sensitive to acoustic overstimulation. Although a threshold shift of 40–70 dB was induced in the untreated ears, the hydropic ears exhibited only a 3–20 dB shift. The other difference was the relation between the amount of threshold shift and the frequency most affected. In the untreated ears, the frequency most affected was above 2 kHz and moved toward the higher frequencies as the threshold shift became larger, although the cochlea was overstimulated by a 2 kHz sound. Considering the amount of the threshold shift, the frequency most affected was much higher in the hydropic ears than the untreated ears (N. Nishikawa, M. Takeyama, J. Kusakari 1990, unpublished data). These results seem to relate to the vibratory patterns of the traveling wave along the basilar membrane. Namely, the maximum amplitude of the vibration moves

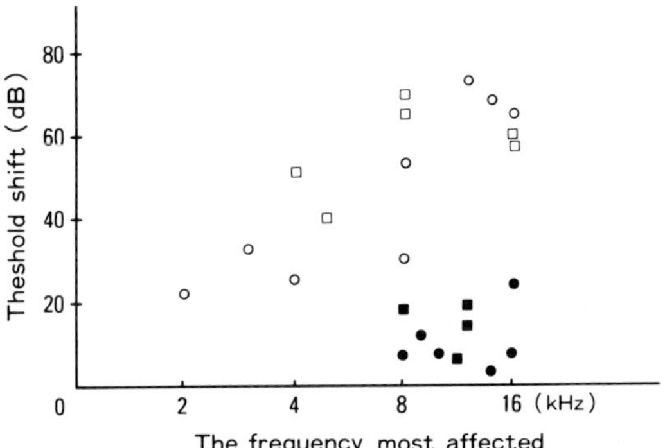

Fig. 5.9. The relation between the frequency most affected in threshold by acoustic overstimulation and the threshold shift of the action potential (AP) at that frequency. Tested at 110 dB(○) and 120 dB(□) sound pressure level (SPL) for 30 min in normal controls and at 110 dB(●) and 120 dB(■) SPL for 30 min in hydropic animals 6 months postoperatively

toward the base of the cochlea with the increase of stimulus strength. Accordingly, the frequency most affected in threshold is higher than that of the overstimulating sound. In the hydropic ears, the traveling wave may dampen earlier due to the volume increment of the endolymph, and the place of the maximum amplitude along the basilar membrane may be shifted toward the more basal portion than in the untreated ears.

Considering the experimental results described in this chapter, the surgically induced hydropic animal is a good animal model of Ménière's disease. Although extensive studies have been performed by many investigators, there are still several discrepancies in opinions and many problems yet to be solved. Further studies with physiological, morphological, biochemical and immunological methods on the hydropic ear induced by other methods as well as the surgical obliteration of the endolymphatic duct and sac will shed light on the pathogenesis of Ménière's disease.

References

1. Harada T (1959) Experimental studies on the disturbance of the circulation of the labyrinthine fluid (in Japanese). J Otolaryngol Jpn 62:319–330
2. Naito T (1959) Clinical and pathological studies on Ménière's disease (in Japanese). J Otolaryngol Jpn 62:2613, 2639–2639
3. Kimura RS (1969) Experimental blockage of the endolymphatic duct and sac and its effect on the inner ear of the guinea pig. Ann Otol Rhinol Laryngol 76:664–687
4. Kusakari J, Arakawa E, Kawase T, Itoh Z, Takeyama M, Rokugo M (1989) Electrophysiological evaluation of the guinea pig with endolymphatic hydrops as an animal model of Ménière's disease. In: Nadol JB (ed) Ménière's disease. Kugler and Ghedini, Amsterdam, pp 267–273
5. Kusakari J, Kobayashi T, Arakawa E, Rokugo M, Ohyama K, Inamura N (1986) Saccular and cochlear endolymphatic potentials in experimentally induced endolymphatic hydrops of guinea pigs. Acta Otolaryngl (Stockh) 101:27–33
6. Kusakari J, Kobayashi T, Arakawa E, Rokugo M, Ohyama K (1987) Time-related changes in cochlear potentials in guinea pigs with experimentally induced endolymphatic hydrops. Acta Otolaryngol [Suppl] (Stockh) 435:27–32
7. Kawase T, Takasaka T, Kusakari J, Shinkawa H, Yuasa R (1989) Effect of external auditory canal pressure upon the hearing threshold in patients with Ménière's disease. Acta Otolaryngol [Suppl] (Stockh) 468:87–92
8. Ito Z, Kusakari J, Kawase T, Takasaka T (1988) Electrocochleographic changes induced by glycerol administration in hydropic guinea pigs (in Japanese). Equilibrium Res [Suppl] 4:54–58
9. Ito Z, Kusakari J, Takeyama M, Nishikawa N, Hara A, Nakata H (1990) The effect of furosemide upon the endocochlear potential in the ear with experimentally induced endolymphatic hydrops. Acta Otolaryngol [Suppl] Stockh (to be published)
10. Konishi T, Kelsey E (1976) Cochlear potentials and electrolytes in endolymph in experimentally induced endolymphatic hydrops of guinea pigs. In: Ruben JR, Elbering C, Salomon G (ed) Electrocochleography. University Park Press, Boston, pp 295–314
11. Konishi T, Salt AN, Kimura RS (1981) Electrophysiological studies of experimentally-induced endolymphatic hydrops in guinea pigs. In: Vosteen K-H, Schuknecht H, Pfaltz CR, Wersäll J, Kimura RS, Morgenstern C, Juhn SK (eds) Ménière's disease: Pathogenesis, diagnosis and treatment. Georg Thieme, New York, pp 47–58
12. Cohen J, Morizono T (1984) Changes in EP and inner ear ionic concentrations in experimental endolymphatic hydrops. Acta Otolaryngol (Stockh) 98:392–402

13. Morgenstern C, Mori N, Amano H (1984) Pathogenesis of experimental endolymphatic hydrops. Acta Otolaryngol [Suppl] (Stockh) 406:56–58
14. Kusakari J, Ise I, Comegys TH, Thalmann I, Thalmann R (1987) Effect of ethacrynic acid, furosemide and ouabain upon the endolymphatic potential and high energy phosphates of the stria vascularis. Laryngoscope 88:12–37
15. Albers FW, de Groot JC, Veldman JE, Huijing EH (1987) Ultrastructure of the stria vascularis and Reissner's membrane in experimental hydrops. Acta Otolaryngol (Stockh) 104:202–210
16. Sellick PM, Johnstone BM (1969) The electrophysiology of the saccule. Pflugers Arch 336:28–34
17. Ninoyu O, Meyer zum Gottesberge AM (1986) Changes in Ca^{++} activity and DC potential in experimentally induced endolymphatic hydrops. Arch Otorhinolaryngol 243:106–107
18. Ikeda K, Kusakari J, Takasaka T (1988) Ionic changes in cochlear endolymph of the guinea pig induced by acoustic injury. Hear Res 32:103–110
19. Klis JF, Smoorenburg GT (1988) Cochlear potentials and their modulation by low-frequency sound in early endolymphatic hydrops. Hear Res 32:175–184
20. Horner KC, Cazals Y (1988) Evoluation of recruitment at different frequencies during the development of endolymphatic hydrops in the guinea pig. Arch Otorhinolaryngol 245:103–107
21. Uno M (1969) Experimental study on the cochlear function in endolymphatic hydrops (in Japanese). J Otolaryngol Jpn 72:1115–1128
22. Kumagami H, Nishida H, Moriuchi M (1981) Changes of the action potential, the summating potential and the cochlear microphonics in experimental endolymphatic hydrops. ORL J Otorhinolaryngol Relat Spec 43:314–327
23. Kumagami H, Miyazaki M (1983) Chronological changes of electrocochleogram in experimental endolymphatic hydrops. Special reference with AP output potential and hair cell cilia. ORL J Otorhinolaryngol Relat Spec 45:143–153
24. Horner KC, Guilhaume A, Cazals Y (1988) Atrophy of middle and short stereocilia on outer hair cells of guinea pig cochleas with experimentally induced hydrops. Hear Res 32:41–48
25. Morizono T, Cohen J, Sikora MA (1985) Measurement of action potential thresholds in experimental endolymphatic hydrops. Ann Otol Rhinol Laryngol 98:191–194
26. van Deelen GF, Ruding PR, Veldman JE, Huizing EH, Smoorenburg GF (1987) Electrocochleographic study of experimentally induced endolymphatic hydrops. Arch Otorhinolaryngol 244:167–173
27. Horner KC, Cazals Y (1987) Rapidly fluctuating thresholds at the onset of experimentally induced hydrops in the guinea pig. Hear Res 26:319–325
28. Takeda T (1981) The electrophysiological study on the hearing loss of Ménière's disease (in Japanese). Pract Otol (Kyoto) 74:2507–2561
29. Martin GK, Shaw DW, Dobie RA, Longsbury-Martin BL (1983) Endolymphatic hydrops in the rabbit: auditory brainstem responses and cochlear morphology. Hear Res 12:65–87
30. Manni JJ, Kuijpers W, Huygen PL, Eggermont JJ (1988) Cochlear and vestibular functions of the rat after obliteration of the endolymphatic sac. Hear Res 36:139–151
31. Aran JM, Rarey KE, Hawkins JE Jr (1984) Functional and morphological changes in experimental endolymphatic hydrops. Acta Otolaryngol (Stockh) 97:547–557
32. Harrison RV, Orsulakova-Meyer zum Gottesberge A, Erre JP, Mori N, Aran JM, Morgenstern C, Tavartkiladze GA (1984) Electrophysiological measures of cochlear function in guinea pigs with long-term endolymphatic hydrops. Hear Res 14:85–91
33. Horner KC, Cazals Y (1988) Independent fluctuations of the round window summating potential and compound action potential following the surgical induction of endolymphatic hydrops in the guinea pig. Audiology 27:147–155
34. Ohashi T, Tomoda K, Yoshie N (1989) Electrocochleographic changes in endolymphatic

hydrops induced by type II collagen immunization through the stylomastoid foramen. Ann Otol Rhinol Laryngol 98:556–562
35. Horner KC, Cazals Y (1987) Glycerol-induced changes in the cochlear responses of the guinea pig hydropic ear. Arch Otorhinolaryngol 244:49–54
36. Long CH III, Morizono T (1987) Hydrostatic pressure measurements of endolymph and perilymph in a guinea pig model of endolymphatic hydrops. Otolaryngol Head Neck Surg 96:83–95

Chapter 6

The Developmental Pattern of Experimental Hydrops in the Endolymphatic Space

Yoshiro Yazawa

Endolymphatic hydrops in the temporal bones of Ménière's disease patients was first described in 1938 by Yamakawa [1] and Hallpike and Cairns [2]. The first successful experimental induction of this condition was by Naito [3] and Kimura and Schuknecht [4], who, in separate studies, produced endolymphatic hydrops in guinea pigs through the obliteration of the endolymphatic duct or sac.

Studies of the developmental patterns of experimental endolymphatic hydrops in guinea pigs have been performed by Kimura and Schuknecht [4], Yanagi [5], Suh and Cody [6], and Ruding et al. [7]. Their respective reports diverge in several respects regarding the stages of hydrops development. Kimura and Schuknecht [4] reported that in the early stages of hydrops development, within the 1st week, cochlear duct dilation was greater in the basal turns, but that in the later stages, after the 3rd week, it became uniform throughout, even appearing more prominent in the higher turns. Yanagi [5] obtained similar results, reporting that 2 days after the obliteration of the sac, dilation was evident in the saccule and in the basal turns of the cochlea, but after 4 weeks was more prominent in the higher turns of the cochlear duct than in the lower. Suh and Cody [6], on the other hand, reported that 1 week after the blockage of the vestibular aqueduct, dilation was evident in the saccule and near the apex of the cohlea duct, and that the dilation usually spread from the apex of the duct to the basal turn in about 2 weeks. Ruding et al. [7] reported that hydrops commenced in the basal coil of the cochlea after about 1 month and proceeded rapidly towards the apex during the 2nd month.

The present study attempted to clarify the developmental patterns of experimental endolymphatic hydrops in guinea pigs through precise measurement of the endolymphatic spaces at various stages of hydrops development, with special attention given to the early stages. Measurements were performed with a light microscope, video camera, and computer arrangement.

An attempt was also made to integrate these animal study results with the established clinical profile of Ménière's disease, in which fluctuating low-tone hearing losses generally characterize the earlier stages, with moderate to severe flat hearing losses gradually coming to predominate during the later stages.

Materials and Methods

Endolymphatic hydrops was induced in guinea pigs using the cauterization method [8, 9], not Kimura's obliteration method [4]. This method, in which the endolymphatic sac was cauterized with silver nitrate, produced consistent endolymphatic hydrops in the animal subjects.

Seventy three healthy female albino guinea pigs were used in this study. After opening the posterior cranial fossa, the right endolymphatic sac was cauterized by injecting a small amount of 10% silver nitrate solution through a micropipette into the sac. The subjects were divided into 8 groups according to their survival time after treatment: 1 day (4 animals), 3 days (8 animals), 1 week (14 animals), 2 weeks (13 animals), 3 weeks (9 animals), 4 weeks (7 animals), 6 weeks (12 animals), and 8 weeks (6 animals). All animals were perfused with normal saline followed by a 10% buffered formaldehyde fixative, after which both ears were removed and kept in an immersion fixation of 10% buffered formaldehyde. The specimens were decalcified in 5% trichloroacetic acid, dehydrated, and embedded using the celloidine-paraffin method. Hematoxylin-eosin stained serial sections were made of the temporal bones.

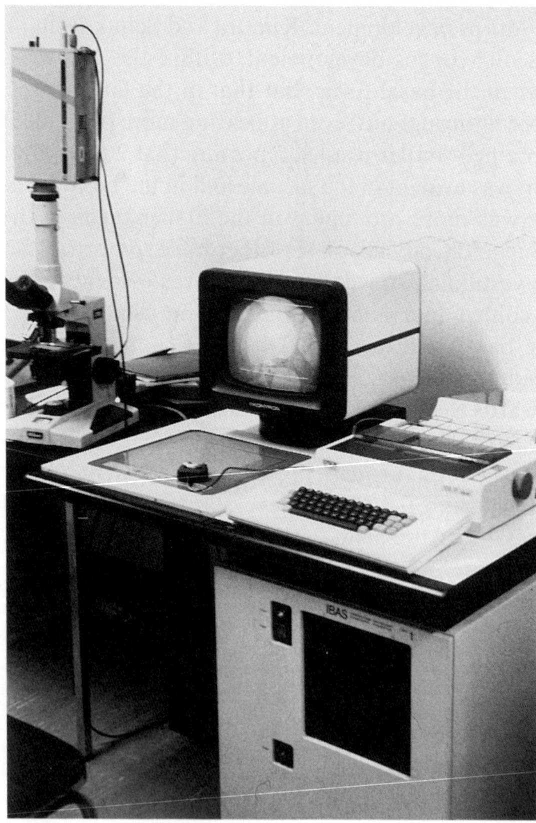

Fig. 6.1. A microscope, video camera, and computer arrangement to measure the endolymphatic space (Kontron IBAS 1 Videoplan)

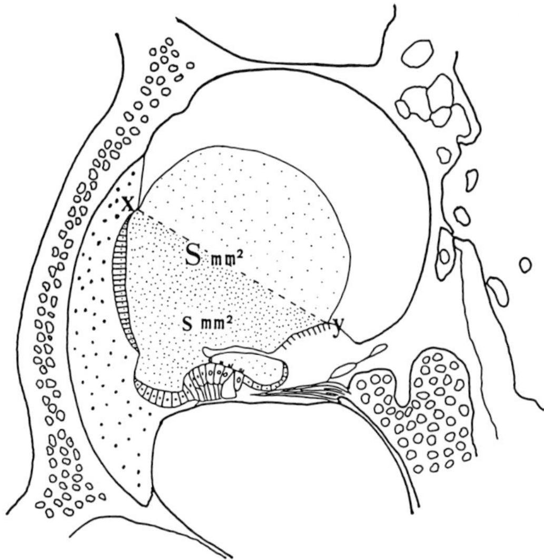

Fig. 6.2. Bulging endolymphatic space (S) and original space of the scala media (s) bounded by *x-y line* of Reissner's membrane. S/s indicates the enlargement ratio of the endolymphatic space

Following the production of temporal bone serial sections, the dilated endolymphatic space (S) and the original endolymphatic space (s) of the saccule, utricle, and each cochlear turn were measured with an arrangement composed of a light microscope, video camera, and computer (Kontron IBAS 1 Videoplan) (Fig. 6.1). The original endolymphatic space, s, served as a control against with the amount of dilatation could be measured. In the utricle and saccule, s was measured using the corresponding section of the left temporal bone, as the left side remained uncauterized and thereby anatomically intact. In the cochlear turn, s was determined by measuring the original scala media space (Fig. 6.2). The enlargement ratio of each endolymphatic space was obtained by dividing S by s and the average enlargement ratio was calculated for the various survival time groups, from 1 day through 8 weeks.

Results

Table 6.1 records the average values for S (the bulging endolymphatic space), s (the original endolymphatic space), and the S/s ratios for the utricle, saccule, and each cochlear turn, classified in groups according to survival time.

In every group the most prominent dilation occurred in the saccule, which steadily expanded to reach a size 6.18 times that of the normal controls at 8 weeks.

The utricle dilated slowly but uniformly to reach a size 2.92 times that of the controls at 8 weeks.

Table 6.1. Endolymphatic space (mm²) and enlargement ratio (S/s) of hydrops

Survival time	Utricle	Saccule	Cochlear turns			
			1st	2nd	3rd	4th
1 days ($n = 4$)						
Hydrops(S)	0.437	0.235	0.086	0.090	0.081	0.075
Control(s)	0.425	0.124	0.080	0.080	0.073	0.070
S/s	1.03	1.89	1.08	1.13	1.11	1.07
3 days ($n = 8$)						
Hydrops(S)	0.487	0.403	0.089	0.086	0.065	0.063
Control(s)	0.363	0.188	0.080	0.076	0.065	0.064
S/s	1.34	2.15	1.11	1.12	0.99	0.98
1 week ($n = 14$)						
Hydrops(S)	0.706	0.416	0.110	0.102	0.095	0.106
Control(s)	0.414	0.134	0.084	0.081	0.071	0.069
S/s	1.70	3.11	1.30	1.25	1.33	1.53
2 weeks ($n = 13$)						
Hydrops(S)	0.603	0.692	0.139	0.144	0.158	0.123
Control(s)	0.335	0.134	0.093	0.085	0.088	0.072
S/s	1.80	5.16	1.49	1.69	1.79	1.71
3 weeks ($n = 9$)						
Hydrops(S)	0.803	0.634	0.136	0.132	0.136	0.122
Control(s)	0.395	0.120	0.082	0.081	0.073	0.064
S/s	2.03	5.28	1.65	1.62	1.86	1.89
4 weeks ($n = 7$)						
Hydrops(S)	0.782	0.838	0.175	0.193	0.144	0.152
Control(s)	0.326	0.149	0.087	0.093	0.077	0.075
S/s	2.39	5.60	2.02	2.07	1.91	2.02
6 weeks ($n = 12$)						
Hydrops(S)	1.108	1.025	0.199	0.199	0.192	0.180
Control(s)	0.422	0.175	0.087	0.088	0.084	0.080
S/s	2.62	5.84	2.29	2.25	2.28	2.25
8 weeks ($n = 6$)						
Hydrops(S)	1.084	0.958	0.205	0.198	0.176	0.156
Control(s)	0.370	0.155	0.084	0.087	0.077	0.069
S/s	2.92	6.18	2.44	2.27	2.29	2.26

The cochlear duct also displayed progressive dilation over the course of the study, but different patterns of development were seen in the respective cochlear turns. One day after cauterization a very slight dilation was seen in all turns. At 3 days, however, the 3rd and 4th turns actually showed a slight shrinkage; the basal turns displayed slight but evident dilation. After 1 week all cochlear turns displayed an almost even degree of hydrops except for the 4th, which showed slightly more dilation than the others. At 2 and 3 weeks, the higher turns exceeded the lower ones in dilation. At 6 weeks, the degree of hydrops was almost the same for all turns, with the S/s value standing at between 2.25 and 2.29. At 8 weeks all cochlear turns except the 1st showed dilation levels nearly the same as those at 6 weeks, with the dilation of the 2nd and 3rd turns being slightly greater than that of the 4th; hydrops in the 1st turn showed a significant increase over the 6-week level, indicating a continuing process of dilation.

Discussion

Several studies have been published to date on the manner in which experimentally induced hydrops develops in the endolymphatic space [4–7]. Common to all of these studies has been the finding that dilation is most prominent in the saccule, followed, in order, by the cochlea and utricle, with no evident dilation observed in the semicircular canals. The reports diverge, however, in their descriptions of hydrops development in the cochlear turns. This divergence may be due in part to such factors as the limited numbers of animals studied, the varying lengths of the respective observation periods, and the approximate nature of the classification systems used, in which the hydrops was defined only as slight, moderate, or profound.

The present study attempted to clarify the nature of hydrops development in guinea pigs through precise measurements of the endolymphatic space at intervals ranging from 1 day to 8 weeks following cauterization of the endolymphatic sac. Particular attention was paid to the cochlear turns.

The present results supported certain of those in earlier studies. The saccule, for example, consistently showed the greatest degree of dilation, reaching (after 8 weeks) a size 6.18 times that of the normal controls. At the end of the study the saccular membrane often touched the footplate of the stapes.

Previous studies have noted varying degrees of dilation for the utricle, but, in general, the amount of hydrops reported has not been high. Kimura and Schuknecht [4] observed less dilation in this structure than in the cochlea, Yanagi [5] noted no evident dilation, and Suh and Cody [6] reported only very slight dilation. The present study discovered profound utricular dilation, however, with the S/s value reaching 2.92 at 8 weeks. This was lower than the degree of hydrops seen in the saccule, but, contrary to the findings of the previous studies, higher than that of the cochlear duct. The low dilation reported in earlier studies may have been due to the manner in which hydrops develops in the utricle. The soft tissue membrane which surrounds this structure allows it to expand quite evenly in all directions, making the degree of dilation appear less than it actually is when judged solely on the basis of visual observation.

At 1 day after the cauterization, all cochlear turns displayed a very slight dilation, with cross-sectional areas ranging from 1.07 to 1.13 times those of the normal controls. At 3 days, however, an actual decrease was seen in the cross-sectional area of the 2 upper turns—to 0.98 and 0.99 times that of the controls—with a slight dilation continuing in the lower turns. The author inferred from this finding that the dilation seen on the 1st day was due to serous labyrinthitis resulting from the surgical and chemical trauma of the cauterization process. Hence, true retention hydrops is considered to have commenced 3 days after cauterization, as the cauterization process requires time to destroy the endolymphatic sac and initiate hydrops formation. The findings at 3 days would thus correspond to the 1st-day findings obtained by Kimura and Schuknecht [4] with the obliteration method, as this method initiated immediate dilation through blockage of the endolymphatic duct.

At 2 and 3 weeks following the cauterization, a greater degree of hydrops was seen in the higher cochlear turns than in the lower. This is consistent with the findings of Kimura and Schuknecht [4] and Yanagi [5], though not with those of Suh and Cody [6] and Ruding et al. [7]. The presence of greater dilation in the higher turns suggests the correspondence of this point in the study with the earlier stages of Ménière's disease, in which fluctuating low-tone hearing losses indicate the involvement of the upper turns of the cochlea.

The more prominent higher-turn dilation apparent in the 2nd and 3rd weeks of this study may be related to the varying lengths of Reissner's membrane in different parts of the cochlear duct. In a previous study [10] it was found that this membrane is longer in the upper turns (0.50–0.55 mm) than in the lower (0.40–0.50 mm), suggesting that the former may be more susceptible to dilation as the endolymphatic pressure increases.

At 4 and 6 weeks after the cauterization, an even degree of hydrops was seen in all cochlear turns, indicating that dilation in the lower turns begins at some point to progress faster than in the upper turns.

At 8 weeks the level of hydrops in the 2nd, 3rd, and 4th turns remained roughly the same as in week 6, but in the 1st turn had increased to a significant degree. The continuing dilation of the 1st turn which this finding demonstrated can be accounted for by the construction of the cochlear duct. By the 8th week the scala vestibuli in the upper turns have no room for further dilation, having expanded to the point where they touch the bony wall. Space still remains in the basal turn, however, allowing for continued bulging as the endolymphatic pressure increases.

These findings suggest that this advanced stage of the study corresponds with the later stages of Ménière's disease, in which nonfluctuating moderate to severe flat hearing loss occurs, indicating involvement of all the cochlear turns.

Summary

The purpose of this experiment was to clarify the pattern of histological change in the inner ear during the development of endolymphatic hydrops. Endolymphatic hydrops was experimentally induced in 73 guinea pigs by the introduction of silver nitrate into the endolymphatic sac. The animals were sacrificed after intervals ranging from 1 day to 8 weeks, and H&E-stained serial sections were made of their temporal bones. The endolymphatic spaces were examined under a light microscope and measured by a computer to determine the pattern of hydrops development. The results were as follows:

1. The saccule displayed the greatest degree of hydrops, dilating up to 6.18 times the size of the saccules in the control group.
2. Cochlear hydrops developed principally in the lower turns during the 1st week, in the upper turns during the 2nd and 3rd weeks, and again in the lower turns during the weeks following. The final result was an even degree of dilation

throughout the cochlea to 2.26–2.29 times normal size, except for the 1st turn, which showed dilation to 2.44 times normal size.

3. The utricle, which has been reported to display minimal dilation, showed a greater dilation than the cochlea—up to 2.92 times normal size.

References

1. Yamakawa K (1938) Über die pathologische Veränderung bei einem Ménière-Kranken. J Otolaryngol Jpn 44:2310–2312
2. Hallpike CS, Cairns H (1938) Observations on the pathology of Ménière's syndrome. J Laryngol 53:625–655
3. Naito T (1959) Clinical and pathological studies on Ménière's disease. In: Proceedings of the 60th annual meeting of the oto-rhino-laryngological society of Japan (in Japanese) 1959, Tokyo, p 46
4. Kimura RS, Schuknecht HF (1965) Membranous hydrops in the inner ear of the guinea pig after obliteration of the endolymphatic sac. Pract Oto-rhino-laryng 27:343–354
5. Yanagi Y (1973) Patterns of hair cell damage of the cochlea due to intense sound stimulation and the cochlear potentials in the guinea pig with experimentally induced endolymphatic hydrops (in Japanese). J Otolaryngol Jpn 76:61–75
6. Suh KW, Cody DT (1974) Obliteration of vestibular and cochlear aqueducts in the guinea pig. Laryngoscope 84:1352–1368
7. Ruding PRJW, Veldman JE, van Deelen GW, Smoorenburg GE, Huizing EH (1987) Histopathological study of experimentally induced endolymphatic hydrops with emphasis on Reissner's membrane. Arch Otorhinolaryngol 244:174–179
8. Yazawa Y (1981) Histopathological study of endolymphatic hydrops (in Japanese). Pract Otol (Kyoto) 74:2450–2506
9. Yazawa Y, Shea JJ, Kitahara M (1985) Endolymphatic hydrops in guinea pigs after cauterizing the sac with silver nitrate. Arch Otolaryngol 111:301–304
10. Yazawa Y, Kitahara M (1989) Elasticity of Reissner's membrane in endolymphatic hydrops (in Japanese). Equilibrium Res [Suppl] 5:96–100

CHAPTER 7

An Animal Model: Ménière's Disease Attack

Kaoru Uchida and Masaaki Kitahara

Endolymphatic hydrops (EH) generally appears to be caused by an imbalance between the secretion and absorption of endolymphatic fluid. Although a model of Ménière's disease has been experimentally produced by inhibiting the absorption of endolymphatic fluid in the endolymphatic sac, it is inappropriate as a model of Ménière's disease since it does not display vertiginous attacks [1–3]. Ménière's attack models have been produced in the past through the use of immunologic reactions [4, 5]. However, such models are considered to be histopathologically different from Ménière's disease, since the existence of considerable precipitation in the perilymphatic spaces indicates the presence of serous labyrinthitis. Kitahara et al. [6] developed a successful Ménière's attack model based on excessive endolymph production by injecting artificial endolymph into the perilymphatic space and the scala media. This fact suggests that excessive endolymph secretion plays a greater role in the occurrence of Ménière's attack than insufficient endolymph absorption.

An attempt was made in this study to create a model of Ménière's attacks by combining excessive endolymph secretion with insufficient endolymph absorption, since the latter factor is incapable of inducing such attacks by itself. Excessive endolymph secretion was induced through the use of histamines (histamine dihydrochloride). Histamines were selected under the consideration that the increased capillary permeability of the stria vascularis which they cause would induce an increased secretion of endolymph. The insufficient endolymph absorption was effected by immunologically obliterating the animals' endolymphatic sacs [3].

Materials and Methods

A total of 101 Hartley guinea pigs weighing 250–450 g were used in this study.

EH was induced with immunologic techniques [3]. Systemic sensitization was performed by the intradermal injection of 1 mg horseradish peroxidase(HRP) in Freund's complete adjuvant. Two injections were made at an interval of 1 week. One week after the second HRP injection, antigen was injected locally into the right endolymphatic sac by opening the posterior cranial fossa according to the method of Kimura and Schuknecht [1].

Histamine was administered intraperitoneally in isotonic saline solution at a level of 20 μg to 1 mg per kilogram of body weight. Histamine administration was performed once at the termination of the experiments, which ranged in length from 1–32 weeks following endolymphatic sac immunization.

The guinea pigs were divided into 3 groups: group A (38 animals), group B (51 animals), and group C (12 animals). Animals in group A underwent both endolymphatic sac immunization and histamine administration. Group B underwent only endolymphatic sac immunization, and those in group C underwent only histamine administration.

The guinea pigs in groups A and B were sacrificed and dissected following intervals of 1–32 weeks after endolymphatic sac immunization. The guinea pigs in group C were sacrificed 1 h after histamine administration.

Spontaneous nystagmus and postural deviation were observed as indications of vestibular function. Spontaneous nystagmus was observed visually; a few animals were also tested with electronystagmographic techniques. Postural deviations were observed with the animals first standing upon a flat surface, then swimming in water with eyes blindfolded. Visual observation of spontaneous nystagmus and postural deviation was performed once a day throughout the experimental period in groups A and B, and for 2 h after histamine administration in groups A and C. Observation of postural deviation during swimming was performed at the termination of the experiment in groups A and C.

Sections were stained with hematoxylin and eosin and studied under the light microscope.

Hydrops in the cochlear duct was graded as 0 (normal), 1 (slight), 2 (moderate), and 3 (profound), in accordance with the classification method of Paparella et al. [7].

Results

The administration of histamines to the 38 guinea pigs in group A caused spontaneous nystagmus attacks in 3 animals and postural deviations on a flat surface in 2 animals. Neither spontaneous nystagmus attacks nor postural deviations were observed in animals in groups B and C. Observation of postural deviations during swimming, however, revealed no significant differences in occurrence rate between groups A and B. Figure 7.1 shows right-beating spontaneous nystragmus in one animal (# 65). The attack occurred 1 h after peritoneal histamine injection (300 μg/kg) 32 weeks after endolymphatic sac immunization. Figure 7.2 shows postural deviation to the left on a flat surface in the same animal.

Figure 7.3 shows the mean $\pm$standard deviation of the degree of EH of all cochlear turns in each group. Animals of group A showed a greater degree of EH than animals of group B. There was a significant difference between the two groups after the 1st week. In group C, only one animal showed a slight EH in the second cochlear turn. Three guinea pigs in which attacks occurred showed profound EH.

In that guinea pig (# 65), which displayed a 2-h attack of spontaneous nystagmus, rupture of Reissner's membrane occurred in the second cochlear turn

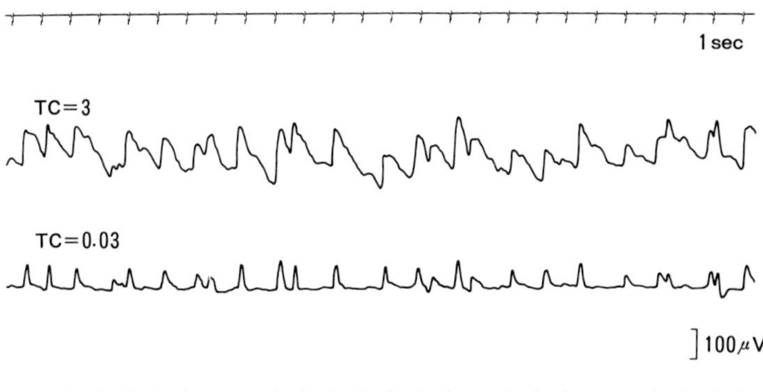

Fig. 7.1. Nystagmus of a guinea pig (# 65). Electrodes were placed on both sides of the right eye to record the horizontal component, and the indifferent electrode was placed on the forehead. Endolymphatic sac immunization was performed in the right ear. Irritable nystagmus is demonstrated. *TC*, time constant

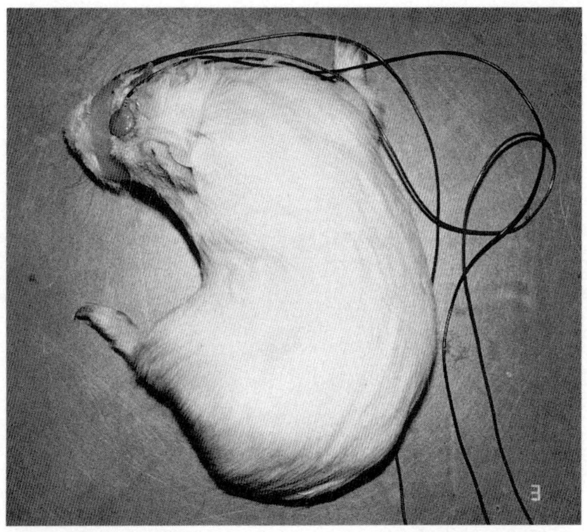

Fig. 7.2. Postural deviation to the left in guinea pig # 65

(Fig. 7.4). In other animals (#s 2, 10) which displayed attacks of a few minutes each, no rupture of Reissner's membrane was detected.

The three guinea pigs which suffered attacks displayed similar severe edema of the stria vascularis. Figure 7.5 shows the stria vascularis of one of them (# 10). Even among the animals in group A which did not experience attacks, a greater occurrence of edema of the stria vascularis was seen than in animals in groups B and C.

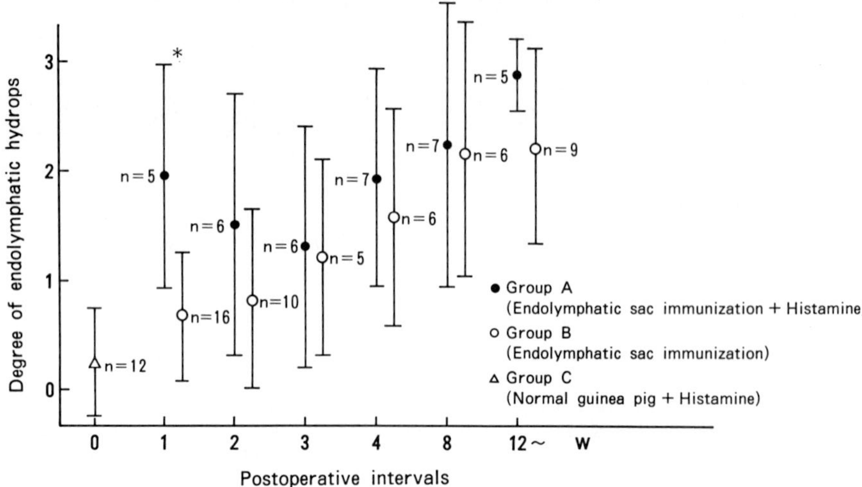

Fig. 7.3. Mean $\pm$ standard deviation of the degree of endolymphatic hydrops (EH) of all cochlear turns in the 3 animal groups. The 12 animals listed at *O* on the horizontal axis belong to group C, the group which received histamine administration alone.* The difference is statistically highly significant, $P < 0.01$; *W*, weeks

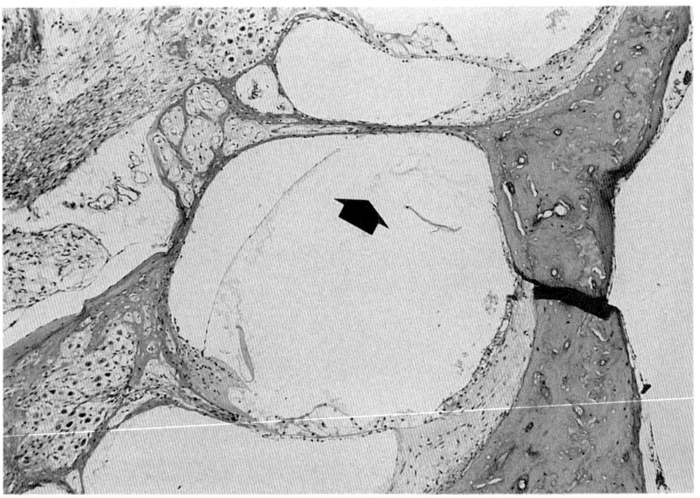

Fig. 7.4. Second cochlear turn of a guinea pig (# 65) which showed ipsilateral nystagmus. Rupture of Reissner's membrane (*arrow*) is present

Discussion

It is generally accepted that the cochlear pathology of Ménière's disease is the distention of Reissner's membrane without any sign of inflammation [8]. Though

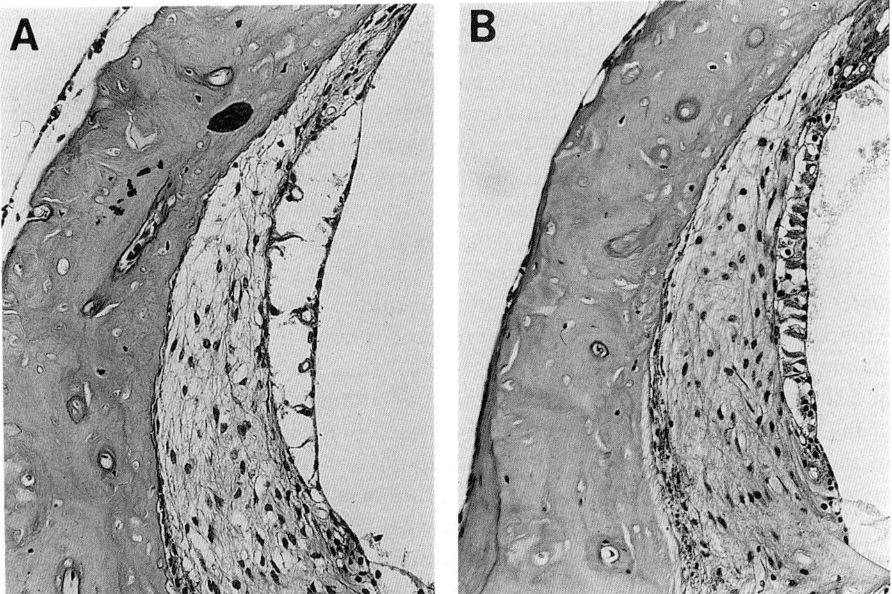

Fig. 7.5A, B. The stria vascularis of the second cochlear turn of a guinea pig that displayed an attack. **A** In the ear with an immunized endolymphatic sac severe edema is shown. **B** In the ear with an untreated endolymphatic sac the stria vascularis is normal

Naito [4] and Hozawa [5] induced Ménière's attacks in guinea pigs utilizing immunologic reactions in the inner ear, the existence of considerable precipitation in the perilymphatic spaces indicated that these models differed histopathologically from the idiopathic EH found in Ménière's patients, as described by Lindsay [8]. A Ménière's attack model showing EH without inflammation in the perilymphatic spaces was successfully produced for the first time in this study.

Concerning the direction of the nystagmus, irritable nystagmus is generally observed early in the attack, followed by a reversal of the nystagmus direction at the end of the attack. Ménière's attacks generally persist from a few minutes to several hours. In this study, two of the three animals which displayed attacks (#s 2, 65) showed nystagmus toward the treated ear, and one (# 10) toward the untreated ear. The nystagmus displayed by the former two animals was similar in form to the nystagmus which occurs during attacks of Ménière's disease. In the latter animal, it may be that irritable nystagmus was not manifested clearly enough to be observable. The direction-changing nystagmus which is usually observed in patients during Ménière's attacks was not observed in these animals. One possible reason for this difference is that paralytic nystagmus was not induced to an observable degree. Further studies of this problem are necessary.

There are at present two theories regarding the direct cause of Ménière's attacks: rapid increase in endolymphatic pressure [9] and rupture of the membranous labyrinth [10, 11]. By perfusing the perilymphatic space with artificial endolymph,

Kitahara et al. revealed experimentally that Ménière's attacks can be caused by either an increase in the potassium concentration of the perilymphatic fluid or an increase in inner ear pressure [6]. In our study, all three guinea pigs which displayed attacks showed profound EH. Rupture of Reissner's membrane (Fig. 7.4) was seen in the second cochlear turn of one guinea pig (# 65), which displayed a 2-h nystagmus attack. This fact suggests that the morphology of the inner ear during Ménière's attacks shows either a marked distention of Reissner's membrane due to an increase in endolymph volume, or a rupture of the membrane itself.

The three animals which displayed attacks all belonged to the group which underwent both endolymphatic sac immunization and histamine administration. Animals of the groups which underwent either one of these two processes did not diaplay attacks. Moreover, guinea pigs in the former group showed a greater degree of EH and edema of the stria vascularis than animals which underwent only one of the two processes. It is reasonable to assume that these alterations were caused by the increased capillary permeability of the stria vascularis induced by histamine action in conjunction with deficient resorption of endolymph in the endolymphatic sac. This experiment suggests that attacks of Ménière's disease are caused by a rapid increase in endolymph pressure due to a rapid rise in endolymph volume and/or an increased concentration of potassium in the perilymphatic spaces caused by the rupture of Reissner's membrane.

Nevertheless, Ménière's attacks were successfully induced in only 3 of the 38 guinea pigs. The Ménière's attacks induced in this experiment may not have been due simply to the addition of the effect of excessive secretion to that of deficient resorption of endolymph. Osako and Hilding [12] reported that endolymph volume did not increase following histamine administration to normal mice. In our study as well, EH was not induced in normal guinea pigs by histamine administration alone, with the exception of a slight degree of hydrops in one animal. Although further study is needed, in view of the fact that animals with attacks displayed severe edema of the stria vascularis, the possibility remains that attacks occurred only in those guinea pigs whose stria vasculari were rendered more susceptible to histamine action through endolymphatic sac immunization without regard to the effects of insufficient endolymph absorption.

References

1. Kimura RS, Schuknecht HF (1965) Membranous hydrops in the inner ear of the guinea pig after obliteration of the endolymphatic sac. Pract Otorhinolaryngol 27:343–354
2. Yazawa Y, Shea JJ, Kitahara M (1985) Endolymphatic hydrops in guinea pigs after cauterizing the sac with silver nitrate. Arch Otolaryngol 111:301–304
3. Sawada I, Kitahara M, Kitajima K, Yazawa Y (1987) Induction of experimental endolymphatic hydrops by immunological techniques. Am J Otol 8:330–334
4. Naito T (1959) Clinical and pathological studies on Ménière's disease (in Japanese). Tokyo, Osaka University, pp 48–49
5. Hozawa J (1980) Immunological consideration recurrent episodes of Ménière's disease (in Japanese). Pract Otol (Kyoto) 73:527–539

6. Kitahara M, Takeda T, Yazawa Y, Matsubara H, Kitano H (1981) Experimental study on Ménière's disease. Otolaryngol Head Neck Surg 90:470–481
7. Paparella MM, Goycoolea MV, Meyerhoff WL (1979) Endolymphatic hydrops and otitis media. Laryngoscope 89:43–54
8. Lindsay JR (1942) Labyrinthine dropsy and Ménière's disease. Arch Otolaryngol 35: 853–867
9. Lindsay JR (1960) Hydrops of labyrinth. Arch Otolaryngol 71:500–510
10. Lawrence M, McCabe BF (1965) Inner-ear mechanisms and deafness: special consideration of Ménière's syndrome. JAMA 171:1927–1932
11. Schuknecht HF, Seifi AE (1963) Experimental observations on the fluid physiology of the inner ear. Ann Otol Rhinol Laryngol 52:687–712
12. Osako S, Hilding DA (1971) Electron microscopic studies of capillary permeability in normal and Ames Waltzer deaf mice. Acta Otolaryngol (Stockh) 71:365–376

CHAPTER 8

An Experimental Study on the Mechanism of the Ménière's Attack: The Influence of High Perilymphatic Potassium Concentration on the Vestibular System

Jiro Hozawa, Keiji Fukuoka, Keiichi Ikeno, Eiji Fukushi, and Koji Hozawa

Clinical characteristics of Ménière's disease are episodic vertigo and fluctuating hearing loss, the origin of which is still obscure. It is well known that nystagmus is always present during the attack, as described by Aschan and Stahle [1], but whose character is not always the same. According to a previous study [2], irritative, paralytic, and reversal nystagmus were observed during the Ménière's attack in 25%, 36%, and 39% of patients, respectively. To explain such complicated clinical manifestations, Schuknecht's membrane rupture theory [3] would be most acceptable. He ascribed the episodic vertigo and fluctuating hearing loss to the rupture and repairing process in the endolymphatic system. His findings were supported by Silverstein [4], who provoked nystagmus by perfusing the perilymphatic space with artificial endolymph. Silverstein thought that sensorineural excitability might be altered by high perilymphatic potassium concentration. Dohlman [5] theorized that, on the basis of the membrane rupture theory, an initial ipsilateral nystagmus could occur due to partial depolarization of the vestibular nerve by the leaking endolymph, and then as the depolarization became more complete, the direction of nystagmus would turn to the contralateral side. Molinari [6] considered that the irritative nystagmus was due to the excitation of the vestibular receptor cells, and that the paralytic nystagmus was due to the inhibitory rebound in the central nervous system. Meissner [7] speculated that the potassium concentration in perilymph determined the extent of depolarization of the sensorineural synpase and brought about the tonus imbalance of the vestibular nuclei followed by ipsi- or contralateral nystagmus. Although these speculations are reasonable explanations for the variation of nystagmus, these theoretical explanations have not been established by clear experimental results.

Therefore, we conducted a study, introducing potassium ion through the round window membrane into the perilymphatic space of guinea pigs, and investigated the influence of the high perilymphatic potassium concentration on the vestibular sensorineural elements and the vestibular nuclei.

Direction Change of the Nystagmus Induced by Introducing Potassium Ions into the Right Perilymphatic Space

In order to elucidate the relation between the direction of nystagmus and vestibular pathology, an animal model of the Ménière's attack was produced on the basis of the membrane rupture theory. At first, 0.2 ml of the saturated solution of potassium chloride was injected into the right tympanic cavities of 60 healthy guinea pigs, and then the iontophoretic procedure was performed for 5 min at 500 μA. Following this procedure, nystagmus which was similar to that of the Ménière's attack was observed. That is, approximately 15 min after the iontophoresis, irritative nystagmus which lasted for about 5 min appeared to the side of the operated ear. After a latent intervals of a few minutes, the second nystagmus developed. At this time, the direction of the nystagmus turned to the contralateral side. Despite the severe attack, this nystagmus was no longer observed on the next day. Electronystagmography showed the directional changing process of nystagmus during this experiment (Fig. 8.1a).

Measurement of Potassium Concentration in Perilymph After Introducing K^+ into the Perilymphatic Space

In order to confirm that the above-mentioned nystagmus was introduced by the high perilymphatic potassium concentration, the following experiment was performed. After dropping a saturated solution of potassium chloride on the round window, the K^+ activity in the perilymph was recorded from the scala tympani of the cochlear basal turn by the double-barrelled K^+ specific microelectrode. As shown in Fig. 8.1b, the perilymphatic potassium concentration began to increase within 1 min after the application, and then a rapid increment was observed. However, this increment of K^+ was not observed by dropping an isoosmotic saccharose solution (Fig. 8.1b). From this result, it was proved that the above-mentioned nystagmus was induced by the high perilymphatic potassium concentra-

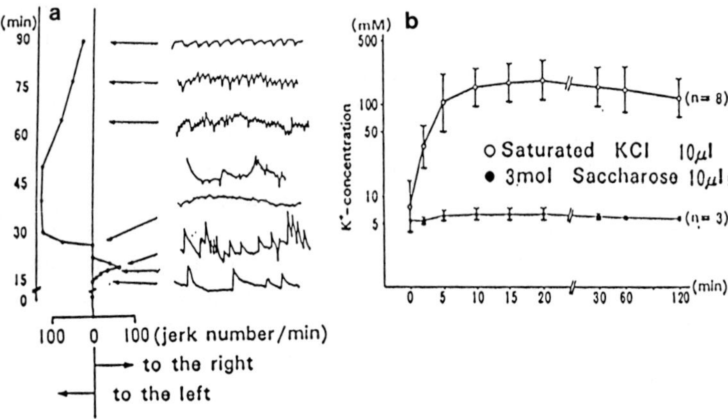

Fig. 8.1. Change of nystagmus and K^+ activity in perilymph after introducing potassium ion into the right perilymphatic space of a guinea pig. **a** Recording of "irritative" and "paralytic" nystagmus. ordinate, the time course after introducing K^+. **b** Recording of K^+ activity in perilymph. abscissa, the time course after introducing K^+

tion. This result corresponded with the result of Silverstein's experiment to support the membrane rupture theory.

Relation Between the Direction of Nystagmus and the Alteration of Vestibular Sensorineural Excitability

Observation of Na-K-ATPase and Succinic Dehydrogenese (SDH) Activity in Vestibular Sensory Cells

The change of sensorineural excitability in the vestibular organ was investigated during the appearance of the above-mentioned nystagmus. Despite the severe nystagmus, no morphological changes of vestibular sensory cells were noticed which seemed to explain the reversible symptoms. On the other hand, enzyme activity of sensorineural elements showed very interesting changes. To observe the enzyme activities, 30 guinea pigs were sacrificed at 10 min, 30 min, 6 h, and 24 h. after introducing potassium ion. Na-K-ATPase was stained by the Mayahara et al.'s one-step lead citrate method [8], and SDH was stained by the Nachlas et al.'s method [9]. At the very early stage of the experiment, as shown in Fig. 8.2a, the

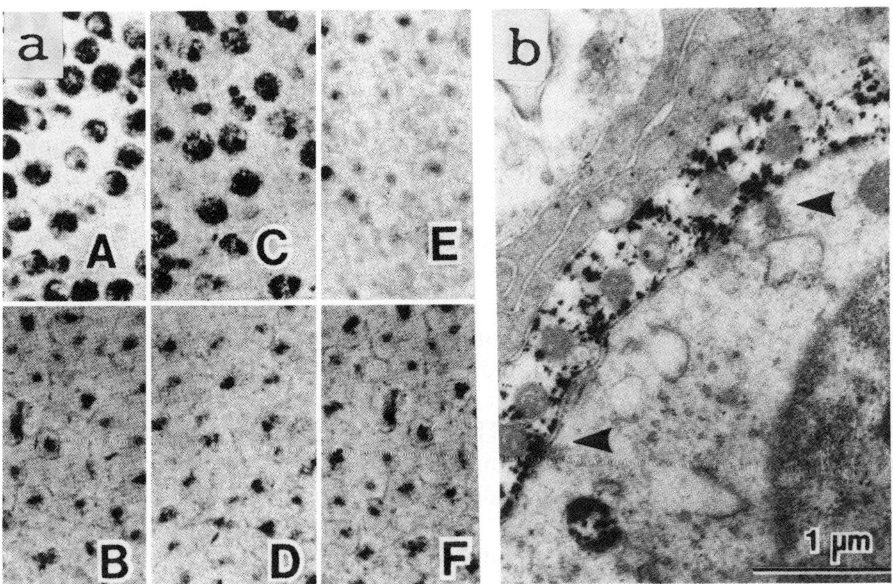

Fig. 8.2a, b. Change of enzyme activity in the vestibular sensory epithelia induced by a high perilymphatic potassium ion concentration **a** Change of SDH activity. SDH in the stage of irritative nystagmus. *A*, operated side and *B*, control side. SDH in the early stage of paralytic nystagmus. *C*, operated side and *D*, control side SDH in the late stage of paralytic nystagmus. *E*, operated side and *F*, control side. **b** Intensive activity of Na-K-ATPase in the irritative nystagmus stage. Precipitates indicating Na-K-ATPase activity are observed in the synaptic area between the sensory cell and the nerve chalice (*arrow*)

SDH activity of the vestibular sensory cells on the operated side was more intensive than that in the non-operated side. This finding was noticed not only during the irritative nystagmus but also in the early stage of paralytic nystagmus. However, in the later stage of paralytic nystagmus, the SDH activity in the vestibular sensory cells on the operated side became weaker than that on the non-operated side (Fig. 8.2a). The Na-K-ATPase activity in the vestibular sensory epithelium showed the same tendency as the SDH activity, and electronmicroscopic observation [10] revealed that the Na-K-ATPase activity was primarily associated with the synpatic area between the vestibular sensory cells and the nerve chalice (Fig. 8.2b).

From these observations, it was concluded that the ipsilateral irritative nystagmus was provoked by the increased excitability of the vestibular sensorineural elements on the operated side, and the contralateral paralytic nystagmus was induced by their decreased excitability. This result seemed to support Dohlman's concept. However, it could not explain the reason why paralytic nystagmus appeared before the decrement of enzyme activity. This delay is thought to be concerned with the central mechanism involving the vestibular nuclei.

Relation Between the Direction of Nystagmus and the Tonus Balance of the Vestibular Nuclei

Autoradiographic Study

To ascertain the possibility that the central regulatory mechanism turns the direction of nystagmus, the glucose uptake of the bilateral vetibular nuclei of 13 guinea pigs was measured during the above-mentioned nystagmus. The [^{14}C]-2-deoxy-D-glucose (2-DG) obtained from New England Nuclea was administrated in a dose of 50 μCi in 0.2 ml sterile saline to the animals, who were sacrificed 45 min after the injection of this radiochemical. The autoradiograph was made by Sokoloff et al.'s method [11], and optical densities of the vestibular nuclei were measured by the microdensitometer (SAKURA) and the computer analyser (OLYMPUS, SP 500). The 2-DG method is widely used to quantify local cerebral glucose consumption; however, the exact measurement of autoradiographic density requires at least 45 min after the injection of 2-DG. Therefore, it is necessary that the irritative as well as the paralytic nystagmus continue up to 45 min. To fullfill this condition, an injection of 0.2 M potassium chloride without the iontophoretic procedure was administered.

As shown in Fig. 8.3, the vestibular nucleus of the operated ear showed the predominant glucose uptake during the appearance of irritative nystagmus, while the contralateral vestibular nucleus showed the predominance during the paralytic nystagmus (Fig. 8.3). The relative values of autoradiographic density in the vestibular nuclei were calculated on the assumption that the density of the adjacent cerebellar hemisphere was 100. The difference in density between the bilateral vestibular nuclei is shown in Table 8.1. The predominant glucose uptake of the ipsilateral vestibular nucleus at the irritative nystagmus stage seems to be due to

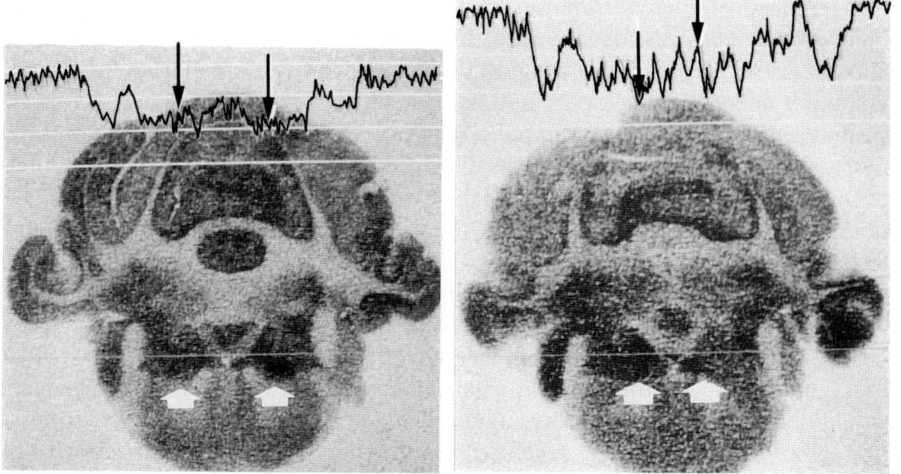

Fig. 8.3a, b. Autoradiograph of the vestibular nuclei by the [^{14}C]-2-deoxy-D-glucose method. *White arrows* indicate left and right vestibular nuclei. Difference in height between two *thin arrows* shows the difference of autoradiographic density. **a** The irritative nystagmus stage. The densitograph recorded in the upper part of this picture shows higher density in the right vestibular nucleus than the left vestibular nucleus. **b** The paralytic nystagmus stage. The density of the left vestibular nucleus is higher than that of the right vestibular nucleus

Table 8.1. Autoradiographic density of vestibular nuclei

Vestibular nuclei	Irritative Stage ($n = 5$)	Paralytic Stage ($n = 5$)
Superior nucleus		
Rt 117.8 ± 6.0[a]	134.0 ± 2.8*	110.9 ± 3.8
Lt 116.8 ± 4.6	117.5 ± 5.0	136.6 ± 2.9*
Lateral nucleus		
Rt 113.6 ± 1.8	119.3 ± 8.3	115.9 ± 3.4
Lt 112.0 ± 1.6	113.2 ± 4.7	135.7 ± 8.0*
Medial nucleus		
Rt 121.9 ± 2.8	138.7 ± 7.3*	122.9 ± 5.6
Lt 122.2 ± 2.6	124.5 ± 7.5	142.5 ± 7.4*
Inferior nucleus		
Rt 111.7 ± 1.9	125.8 ± 2.1*	111.6 ± 4.0
Lt 110.0 ± 3.7	114.7 ± 6.3	135.8 ± 4.4*

The relative values were calculated on the assumption that the density of the adjacent cerebellar hemisphere is 100. The higher density of the right vestibular nucleus is observed at the irritative nystagmus stage, and the left vestibular nucleus shows higher density at the paralytic nystagmus stage.

*$p < 0.05$

[a] Numbers in *parentheses* are the normal values

the increment of afferent impulse, which was induced by the sensorineural excitations on the operated-side labyrinth. In the same experimental models as ours, T Kawase (1986) recorded the change of single unit action potential from the superior vestibular nerve of guinea pigs, and concluded that "irritative nystagmus" could be induced by the increased impulse of the vestibular nerve and the "paralytic nystagmus" could be ascribed to the disappearance of the nerve activity.

On the other hand, the predominant glucose uptake of the contralateral vestibular nucleus, which was noticed at the paralytic nystagmus stage, was thought to be caused by the impulse from the non-operated side labyrinth, and its effect would be manifested by the release of commissural inhibition [12] in the vestibular nucleus of the operated side. It should be noticed that the several of glucose uptake between the bilateral vestibular nuclei corresponded with the onset of paralytic nystagmus. Namely, the tonus imbalance between the bilateral vestibular nuclei would decide the direction of nystagmus. Therefore, the reason why the paralytic nystagmus began to appear, despite the continuing sensorineural excitation of the labyrinth, would be explained by this experimental result which seems to support Meissner's speculation.

Conclusion

From the results of our experiments, it was concluded:

1. The membrane rupture theory is a reasonable explaination of the mechanism of the Ménière's attack.
2. A high perilymphatic potassium concentration induced by the rupture of the membranous labyrinth would provoke the irritative as well as the paralytic nystagmus.
3. The direction of nystagmus during the Meniere's attack is related to the vestibular sensory cells' excitability. Namely, irritative nystagmus is provoked by increased excitability, and paralytic nystagmus is concerned with decreased excitability.
4. However, the direction of nystagmus is ultimately decided by the tonus imbalance between the bilateral vestibular nuclei, which is induced by the difference of sensorineural excitability between both labyrinths.

References

1. Aschan G, Stahle J (1957) Nystagmus in Ménière's disease during attacks. Acta Otolaryngol (Stockh) 47: 189–201
2. Hozawa J, Fukuoka K, Usami S, Kamimura T, Hozawa K (1986) Experimental studies on mechanism of the Ménière's attack (in Japanese). Auris Nasus Larynx 13 (Suppl II): 21–27
3. Schuknecht HF (1963) Ménière's disease; a correlation of symptomatology and pathology. Laryngoscope 73: 651–665
4. Silverstein H (1970) The effect of perfusing the perilymphatic space with artificial endolymph. Ann Otol Rhinol Laryngol 79: 754–765

5. Dohlman GF (1980) Mechanism of the Ménière's attack. ORL J Otorhinolaryngol Relat Spec 42:10–19
6. Molinari GA (1972) Alterations of inner ear mechanism resulting from application of sodium chloride to the round window membrane. Ann Otol Rhinol Laryngol 81:315–323
7. Meissner R (1981) Behavior of the nystagmus in Ménière's attack. Arch Otorhinolaryngol 223:173–177
8. Mayahara H, Fujimoto K, Ogawa K (1980) A new one-step method for the cytochemical localization of ouabain-sensitive potassium dependent *p*-nitrophenyl phosphate activity. Histochemistry 67:125–138
9. Nachlas MM, Tsou KC, Souza F, Seligman AM (1957) Cytochemical demonstration of succinic dehyrogenese by the use of a new *p*-nitrophenyl substituted ditetrasole. J Histochem Cytochem 5:420–436
10. Hozawa K, Takasaka T, Fukuoka K, Usami S, Hozawa J (1987) Effect of high perilymphatic potassium concentration on the guinea pig vestibular sensory epithelium. Acta Otolaryngol [Suppl] (Stockh) 435:21–26
11. Sokoloff L, Reirich M, Kennedy C (1977) The [^{14}C] deoxyglucose method for the measurement of local cerebral glucose utilization: Theory, procedure, and normal values in the conscious and anesthetized albino rat. J Neurochem 28:897–916
12. Mano N, Oshima T, Shimazu H (1968) Inhibitory commissural fibers interconnecting the bilateral vestibular nuclei. Brain Res 8:378–382

CHAPTER 9

A Pathohistological Study with Four Kinds of Stress Stimulations on Active Endolymphatic Hydrops in Guinea Pigs

Katsuya Akioka, Yoshiyuki Kitaoku, Osamu Tanaka, and Takashi Matsunaga

Ménière's disease is believed to show pathological features of endolymphatic hydrops [1, 2], but the etiology of this disease has not yet been ascertained. Many investigators [3], have attempted to create animal models with endolymphatic hydrops by obliterating the endolymphatic sac and duct. However, this method has been unable to adequately explain the development of Ménière's disease because it uses simulated apparatus. On the other hand, Ménière's disease is thought to develop as a result of stress to the inner ear mechanism although there have been no reports on endolymphatic hydrops induced by stress. We conducted a short-term experiment, creating active endolymphatic hydrops by stress load, to study the occurrence rate of endolymphatic hydrops. This was followed by a light-microscopic study on the changes in permeability of the cochlear lateral wall with horseradish peroxidase and a study of the dynamics of endolymphatic hydrops.

Materials and Methods

Experiment to Study the Occurrence Rate of Active Endolymphatic Hydrops

We used 48 white guinea pigs weighing 300–600 g. All of the guinea pigs showed normal Preyer's reflex. First, under local anesthesia with xylocaine, we sympathectomized the left stellate ganglion of the animals to cause autonomic imbalance and then strangulated the left carotid artery to create a circulation disorder of the inner ear. Then, Compound 48/80 (1 mg/kg) was injected intraperitoneally to cause hyperpermeability in the vessels of the inner ear. Finally, the animals were exposed to 2 h of 130 dB of white noise (Nagashima type PA-1) as stress load. All the animals were then perfused with Wittmaack fixative solution, and both inner ears were surgically removed, fixed with Wittmaack solution, decalcified, dehydrated, embedded with celloidin, and stained with hematoxylin eosin solution. As the last step in the experiment, we examined the occurrence rate of endolymphatic hydrops in these animals.

Experiment to Study Changes in Permeability of the Cochlear Lateral Wall

The animals were divided into 2 groups: stress group (3 animals) and untreated group (3 animals). We conducted the experiment to examine changes in permeability of the lateral cochlear wall by stress-loading with horseradish peroxidase (HRP, Sigma type II, M.W. 40,000, radius 25Å). Horseradish peroxidase (25,000 units in a 1-ml saline solution) was slowly injected into the jugular vein by catheterization. Five minutes after injection perfusion with a solution of 2% glutaraldehyde and 1% paraformaldehyde and then surface preparation were performed. Next, the dissected tissues were stained with 0.1% 3,3′-diaminobenzidine tetrahydrochloride and routinely dehydrated, embedded in paraffin and counterstained with hematoxylin. The tissue-slides were then light microscopically studied.

Results

Experiment to Study the Occurrence Rate of Active Endolymphatic Hydrops

Altogether, 42 right cochleae and 37 left cochleae were suitable for histological evaluation. The occurrence rate of active endolymphatic hydrops of the right cochlea was 33.3% and that of the left cochlea was 37.8%. It was more frequent on the sympathectomized side of the stellate ganglion than on the nonsympathectomized side (Table 9.1). Endolymphatic hydrops was found to occur frequently in the basal and second turns (Table 9.2). Most of the incidents of endolymphatic hydrops were associated with the nubecula in the scala vesibuli (Figs. 9.1, 9.2). At higher magnification of the same specimens, we could see no remarkable changes in either the stria vascularis or the organ of Corti (Fig. 9.3).

Table 9.1. The occurrence rate of hydrops

Left cochlea ($n = 37$)	37.8%
Right cochlea ($n = 42$)	33.3%

Table 9.2. The distribution rate of hydrops in the cochlea

	Turn affected (%)			
Cochlea	Basal	Second	Third	Apical
Left ($n = 37$)	10.8%	21.6%	5.4%	2.7%
Right ($n = 42$)	21.4%	19.0%	4.8%	7.1%

Experiment to Study Changes in Permeability of the Cochlear Lateral Wall

In all cases of untreated control animals, horseradish peroxidase was distributed only in and around the vessels, in both the stria vascularis and the spiral ligament (Fig. 9.4). In all cases of the animals of the stress group, horseradish peroxidase was present throughout the stria vascularis, while in the spiral ligament, it was

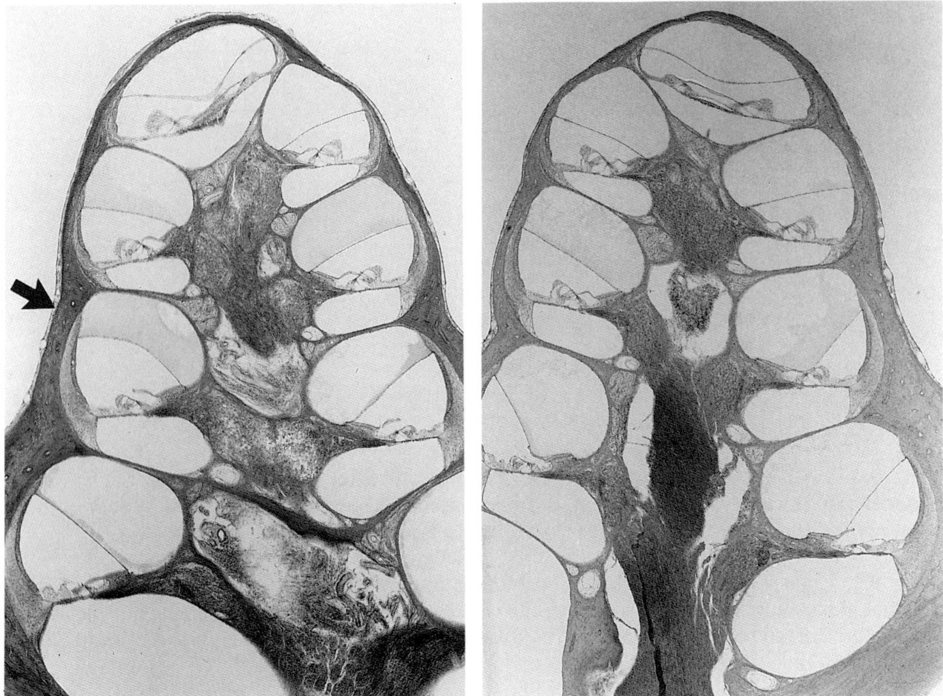
9.1 9.2

Fig. 9.1. Light micrograph of the left cochlea after stress stimulation. Hydrops is shown (*arrow*) in the second turn (H & E stain, × 5)

Fig. 9.2. Light micrograph of the right cochlea of the guinea pig in Fig. 9.1 after stress stimulation. No hydrops is present (H & E stain, × 5)

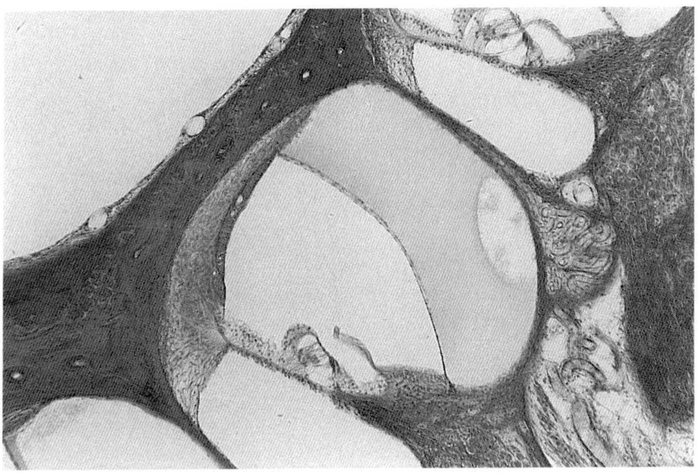

Fig. 9.3. High magnification of the second turn of the cochlea in Fig. 9.1. Neither atrophy in the stria vascularis nor abnormality in the organ of Corti can be seen (H & E stain, × 20)

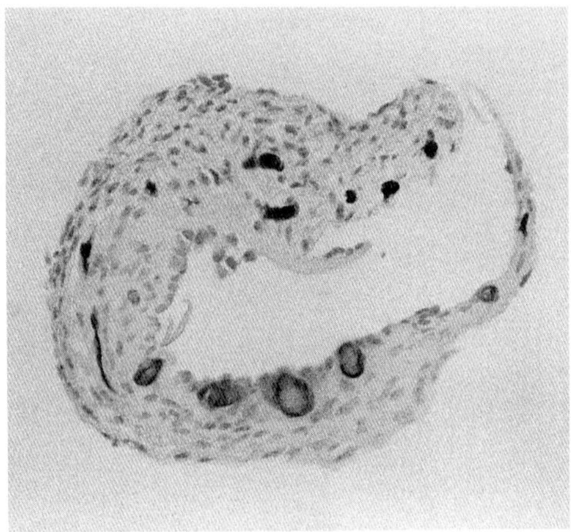

9.4

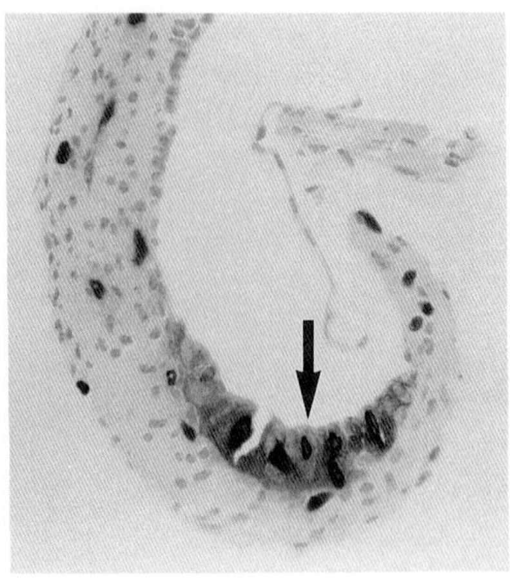

9.5

Fig. 9.4. Light micrograph of the cochlear lateral wall after HRP injections in the control guinea pig. Both the spiral ligament and stria vascularis show reaction products only in the vessels and their surrounding areas (DAB reaction and hematoxylin stain, × 100)

Fig. 9.5. Light micrograph of the left cochlear lateral wall after stress stimulation. The spiral ligament has reaction products only in the vessels and their surrounding areas, but the stria vascularis (*arrow*) clearly contains diffuse reaction products (DAB reaction and hematoxylin stain, × 100)

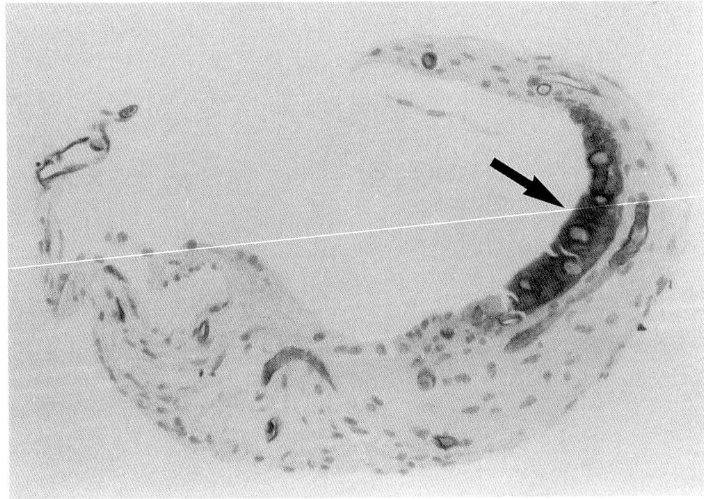

Fig. 9.6. Light micrograph of the right cochlear lateral wall after stress stimulation. Reaction products (*arrow*) are similar to those in Fig. 9.5 in terms of localization and quality (DAB reaction and hematoxylin stain, × 100)

distributed only in and around the vessels (Figs. 9.5, 9.6). Our experiment did not show that changes in permeability on the sympathectomized side were more significant than those on the nonsympathectomized side.

Discussion

Naito [4] reported that it was difficult to cause endolymphatic hydrops with a single stimulation. However, in both Naito's and our experiments, it was shown that several stimulations could cause endolymphatic hydrops, perhaps because several stimulations had enough energy to cause endolymphatic hydrops. The endolymphatic hydrops of our experiment was rather mild with a low incidence rate. In this sense, it resembled human endolymphatic hydrops, which also tends to be mild. Endolymphatic hydrops was more frequent on the sympathectomized side of the stellate ganglion than on the nonsympathectomized. This showed that sympathectomization contributed to the development of endolymphatic hydrops with regard to the enlargement of vessels. In our present experiment, endolymphatic hydrops was found to be most frequent in the basal and second turns, which is contrary to the characteristic hearing loss in the low-pitched sound area associated with Ménière's disease. The reason for this discrepancy remains unclear. Sakagami et al. [5] reported that vessel permeability in the stria vascularis was highly changeable, while that in the spiral ligament was not. We obtained the same results with stress stimulations in this experiment. It was therefore assumed that increased permeability of the stria vascularis vessels was one of the causes of endolymphatic hydrops. We plan to study the development mechanism of endolymphatic hydrops in relation to the endolymphatic sac and duct.

Summary and Conclusion

We administered 4 types of stress stimulation to guinea pigs and studied the occurrence rate of active endolymphatic hydrops and changes in the permeability of the cochlear lateral wall. Endolymphatic hydrops occurred at a low rate and was relatively mild. The development of endolymphatic hydrops occurred more frequently on the sympathectomized side of the stellate ganglion than on the nonsympathectomized side. Endolymphatic hydrops was most frequent in the basal and second turns. In response to the stress stimulations of the present experiment, permeability of the spiral ligament hardly increased, while that of the stria vascularis increased appreciably. It is assumed that increased permeability of the vessels of the stria vascularis was one of the causes of endolymphatic hydrops.

References

1. Yamakawa K (1938) Über die pathologische Veränderung bei einem Ménière-Kranken. J Otolaryngol Jpn 44:2310–2312

2. Hallpike CS, Cairns H (1938) Observations on the pathology of Ménière's syndrome. J Laryngol Otol 53: 625–655
3. Kimura RS (1976) Experimental pathogenesis of hydrops. Arch Otorhinolaryngol 212: 263–275
4. Naito T (1973) Ménière's disease (in Japanese). Pract Otol (Kyoto) 66: 1–50
5. Sakagami M, Matsunaga T, Hashimoto PH (1982) Ultrastructural study on the permeability of blood vessels in the inner ear: Capillaries of the stria vascularis and spiral ligament (in Japanese). Practica Otol (Kyoto) 75: 2451–2458

Chapter 10

The Effect of Steroids on Endolymphatic Hydrops Induced by an Immunological Technique

Yoshiro Yazawa, Masaaki Kitahara, Kaoru Uchida, and Izumi Sawada

Steroids are less frequently used for the treatment of Ménière's disease compared with their use for sudden deafness or facial paresis. Hauser [1] reported 2 cases of Ménière's disease in which hearing was improved by the administration of steroids. McCabe [2], Hughes et al. [3, 4] and Shea [5] also reported the efficacy of steroids in cases of sensorineural hearing loss and/or Ménière's disease with a suspected immunological origin. According to our 1970 and 1980 nationwide surveys [6, 7], incidences where otolaryngologists treated Ménière's disease with steroids increased from 2% to 7%. It is true that steroids are one of the few drugs which have promising effects on certain types of Ménière's disease. This study was made to examine the effects of steroids on endolymphatic hydrops experimentally induced in guinea pigs by an immunological technique [8].

Materials and Methods

Fifty female Hartley guinea pigs with positive Pryer's reflex, weighing 200–350 grams, were used in this study. The antigen used for the immunization was horseradish peroxidase (HRP). An emulsion was made by adding 1 mg of HRP dissolved in 0.5 ml of normal saline to an equal amount of Freund's complete adjuvant and then homogenizing the mixture. The guinea pigs received intradermal injection of 1 mg of HRP emulsified with Freund's complete adjuvant. All guinea pigs were given a booster once more with an identically prepared emulsion after 1 week. One week after the booster, local immunization was achieved by opening the posterior cranial fossa, inserting a micropipette into the right endolymphatic sac, and injecting a small amount (0.01 ml) of identical emulsion with a microsyringe [8]. The guinea pigs were divided into 3 groups; A(n = 10), B(n = 10), and C(n = 10). In group A, immediately after local immunization, 10 animals started to receive 5 intraperitoneal injections of betamethasone (1 mg each time) at 7-day intervals. In group B, 3 weeks after local immunization 10 animals started to receive 5 injections of the same amount of betamethasone at 5-day intervals. Group C did not receive betamethasone after local immunization. All these guinea pigs were sacrificed for histological examination 6 weeks after local immunization. The hearing thresholds of these guinea pigs were examined by means of electrocochleography (click sound) immediately before sacrifice. The protocol of this experiment is shown in Fig. 10.1.

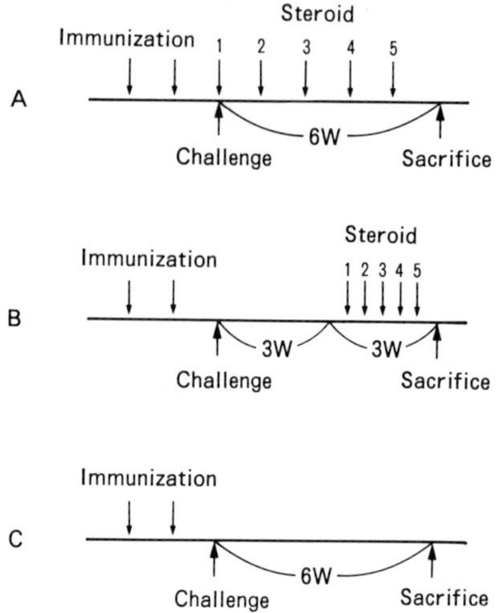

Fig. 10.1. Protocol of the experiment

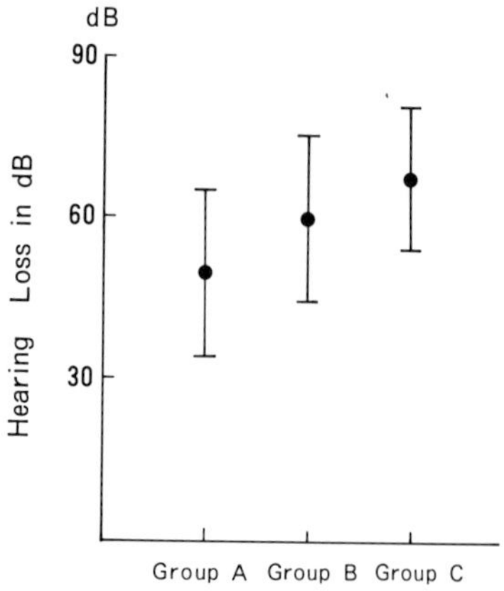

Fig. 10.2. Averaged hearing thresholds in groups A, B, and C. Bars indicate standard deviation.

Another group of 20 animals was used for the histological examination of the endolymphatic sacs anywhere from 3 hours to 2 weeks after local immunization. In 11 out of 20 animals, betamethasone was injected 3–5 times immediately before and/or after local immunization. Betamethasone was not administrated to the other 9 animals.

Serial sections of the temporal bones were stained with hematoxylin-eosin, and the degree of hydrops in the 3 groups was examined under a light microscope and then compared. The endolymphatic sacs were also carefully examined, especially with regard to the degree of cell infiltration and to the formation of soft granulation.

Results

Averaged hearing thresholds of groups A, B, and C with standard deviations are shown in Fig. 10.2. Averaged hearing thresholds became higher, with group C being more affected than group A. The difference in the averaged thresholds between group A and C was significant.

The degree of hydrops in each cochlear turn was scored according to Paparella et al.'s classification [9]. Mean averaged scores of all cochlear turns of groups A, B and C, with standard deviations, are shown in Fig. 10.3. The mean averaged scores of all cochlear turns became smaller from C to B to A, with that of group A being significantly less than that of group C.

Hydrops of the saccule was classified into 3 grades. The mean score of the saccules of groups A and B were significantly less than that of group C (Fig. 10.4).

The endolymphatic sacs which received immunological challenge with HRP were replaced by soft granulation. No significant difference was noted in the grade of formation of granulation 6 weeks after local immunization among groups A, B,

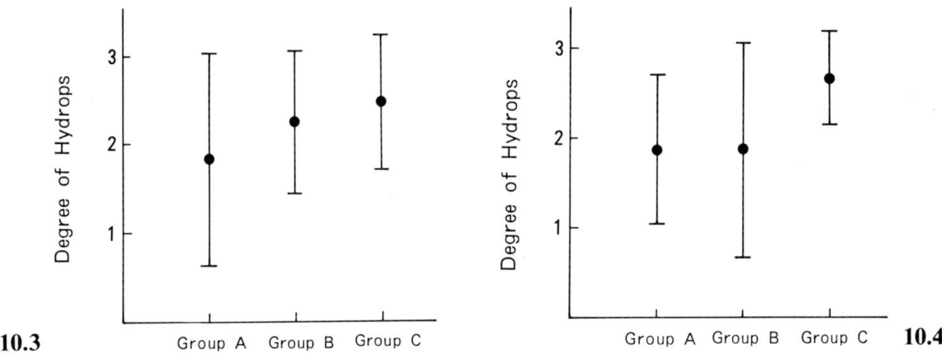

Fig. 10.3. Mean averaged hydrops scores of all cochlear turns in groups A, B, and C. Bars indicate standard deviation.

Fig. 10.4. Mean hydrops scores of saccules in groups A, B, and C. Bars indicate standard deviation.

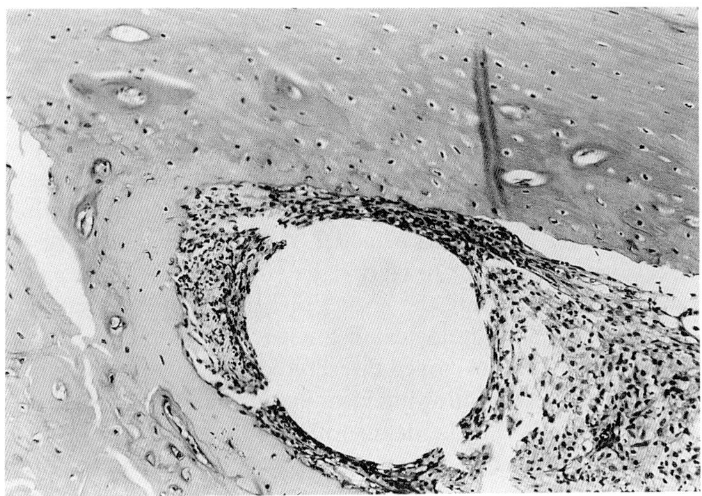

Fig. 10.5. Formation of endolymphatic sac granulation 1 week after local immunization of a guinea pig which received batamethasone. Formation of granulation is inhibited. Sac cavity remains open.

and C. However, the formation of granulation was slighter in animals which received betamethasone (Fig. 10.5) than in the control animals (Fig. 10.6), 1–2 weeks after local immunization. Infiltration of monocytes and neutrophils was also more inhibited in animals with betamethasone administration than in the control animals, 1–3 days after local immunization.

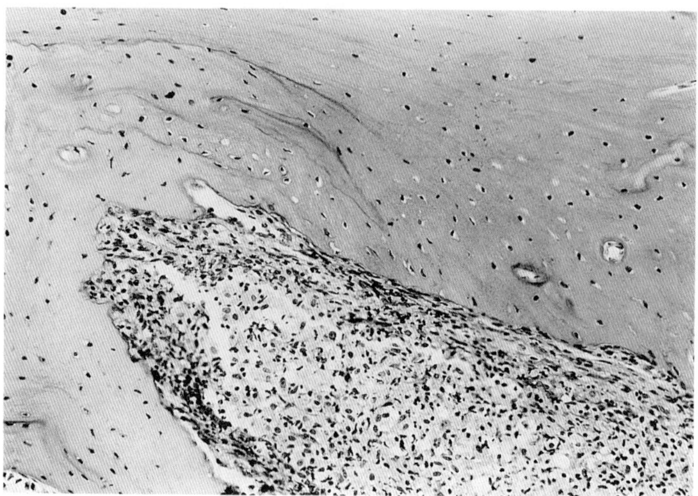

Fig. 10.6. Formation of endolymphatic sac granulation 1 week after local immunization of guinea pig which did not receive betamethasone. Sac cavity is completely obliterated by granulation.

Discussion

In a previous report [8], we succeeded in inducing endolymphatic hydrops in 65% of the guinea pigs by means of the immunological technique. Although the figure of 65% was less than that obtained by Kimura and Schuknecht's method [10], this type of hydrops could be used as a model of Ménière's disease of one type of immunological origin. In order to clarify the efficacy of steroids on this type of Ménière's disease, in this study the effects of betamethasone on endolymphatic hydrops induced by an immunological technique were examined.

It was revealed that 1) the averaged threshold of hearing of guinea pigs receiving betamethasone immediately following local immunization was significantly lower than that in the controls. 2) The degree of hydrops was reduced in guinea pigs which received betamethasone immediately following local immunization and 3 weeks after local immunization. The difference in the degree of hydrops was significant between the controls and the guinea pigs which received betamethasone immediately following local immunization. 3) The grade of hydrops in the saccules of guinea pigs which received betamethasone was significantly smaller than that of the controls. 4) No difference was observed in the grade of formation of granulation in the endolymphatic sacs among all groups 6 weeks after local immunization.

In this study of guinea pigs which received betamethasone, no folding of Reissner's membrane was observed although the degree of hydrops was less than that in the controls. According to Kimura [11], in guinea pigs with endolymphatic hydrops induced by mechanical obliteration of the endolymphatic sac and duct, suppression of endolymphatic hydrops by the application of steroids was not observed. In this study, therefore, betamethasone is considered to effect the endolymphatic sac at an early stage following local immunization. In fact, as shown in Figs. 10.5 and 10.6, formation of granulation was markedly depressed 1–2 weeks following local immunization in cases where betamethasone was administered. In a previous study [12], it was proven that endolymphatic pressure slightly exceeded perilymphatic pressure at this early stage, but that they became almost equal afterwards. Kawase et al. [13] reported that the hearing threshold was decreased by applying pressure to the perilymphatic fluid at an early stage of the development of hydrops, but increased by the same pressure at a later stage. These facts seem to agree with the results shown in this study—that an early administration of betamethasone is more effective than a later administration.

This model of Ménière's disease is only one type of the disease associated with an immunological process. It is difficult to generalize the facts obtained from this study to include every type of Ménière's disease of immunological origins. However, steroids such as betamethasone are considered to be effective for a certain type of Ménière's disease, especially when applied at an early stage.

References

1. Hauser E (1959) Ménière's disease; a new therapeutic approach. J Am Geriatr Soc 7:874–876
2. McCabe BF (1979) Autoimmune sensorineural hearing loss. Ann Otol Rhinol Laryngol 88:585–589
3. Hughes GB, Kinney SE, Barna BP, Calabrese LH (1983) Autoimmune reactivity in Ménière's disease. A preliminary report. Laryngoscope 93:410–417
4. Hughes GB, Barna BP, Kinney SE, Calabrese LH, Hamid MA, Nalepa NJ (1988) Autoimmune endolymphatic hydrops: five-year review. Otolaryngol Head Neck Surg 88:221–225
5. Shea JJ (1983) Autoimmune sensorineural hearing loss as aggravating factor in Ménière's disease. Adv Otorhinolaryngol 30:254–257
6. Yagi N, Kitahara M (1972) Treatment for Ménière's disease (in Japanese). Pract Otol (Kyoto) 65:923–930
7. Kitajima K, Saito H, Kitano H, Kitahara M (1981) The trend of treatment in Ménière's disease during the past 10 years (in Japanese). Pract Otol (Kyoto) 74:2396–2405
8. Sawada I, Kitahara M, Kitajima K, Yazawa Y (1987) Induction of experimental endolymphatic hydrops by immunologic technique. Am J Otol 8:330–334
9. Paparella MM, Goycoolea MV, Meyerhoff WL, Shea D (1979) Endolymphatic hydrops and otitis media. Laryngoscope 89:43–54
10. Kimura RS, Schuknecht HF (1965) Membranous hydrops in the inner ear of the guinea pig after obliteration of the endolymphatic sac. Pract Oto-rhino-larying 27:343–354
11. Kimura RS (1985) Surgical and drug intervention in experimentally induced endolymphatic hydrops. In: Nomura Y (ed) Hearing and dizziness. Igaku-Shoin, Tokyo, p 16
12. Matsubara H (1981) Basic experiment of attacks of Ménière's disease (in Japanese). Pract Otol (Kyoto) 74:2418–2449
13. Kawase T, Kusakari J, Shinkawa H, Takasaka T (1988) Effect of perilymphatic pressure on the CM threshold in hydropic ears of guinea pigs (in Japanese). Equilibrium Res [Suppl] 4:37–40

CHAPTER 11

A Pathoanatomical Study of the Endolymphatic Sac in Ménière's Disease

Yoshiro Yazawa and Masaaki Kitahara

It has been well established by anatomic and tomographic reports [1, 2] that the endolymphatic sac (ELS) and vestibular aqueduct (VA), appear in great varieties of size, position, course, and form. These irregularities are particularly pronounced in Ménière's disease, with tomographic studies revealing the VA to be filiform, stenotic, or nonvisualized in more than 50% of all Ménière's cases [3, 4]. Such tomographic findings were used by Stahle and Wilbrand [4, 5] in the development of a system classifying the degree of peri-aqueductal pneumatization in Ménière's disease into 3 grades: large cell pneumatization, small pneumatization, and non-pneumatization.

Variations in the size, position, and vascularity of the sacs in Ménière's disease have also been observed during ELS surgery. Shambaugh [2] and House [6], for example, reported that the ELS could not be identified in 10%–14% of patients with Ménière's disease during sac operations. Shambaugh et al. [7] also reported ischemia of the exposed wall of the ELS and the partial or complete obliteration of the lumen of the sac in the majority of Ménière's disease cases. These surgical findings were utilized by Arenberg et al. [8] in their modification of Stahle's tomography-based grading system into a new group with three classifications, labeled type I, type II, and type III respectively.

Such characteristics as the position, size, and vascularity of the ELS in Ménière's disease are examined in the above surgical reports, but their findings are limited to the subjective observations of the surgeon; no statistical studies of these characteristics or comparisons with non-Ménière's disease ELSs were performed. The present study is an attempt to address these issues through a statistical examination of the position, size, color, and vascularity of the sacs in 46 cases of Ménière's disease, and a subsequent comparison of the results with those obtained in 12 cases of non-Ménière's disease.

Materials and Methods

The present study utilized the photographs and surgical records of 46 patients with Ménière's disease who underwent ELS drainage surgery [9] between 1984–1987. The photographs of the exposed endolymphatic sacs were taken from several

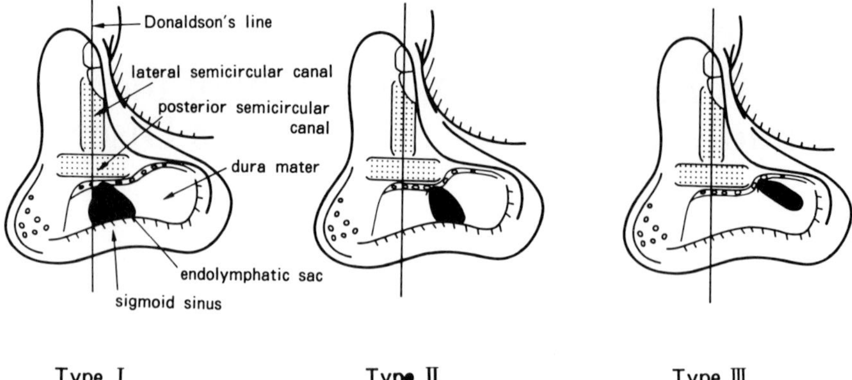

Fig. 11.1. Anatomical classification of the endolymphatic sac position: *type I*, *II* and *III* (modified from Arenberg et al.'s classification [8]).

angles and at various magnifications. The materials were examined to obtain pathoanatomical data on the position, size, surface color, and vascularity of the ELSs. These data were then used to categorize the sacs with regard to each of the 4 characteristics studied.

The control study was based on the photographs and surgical records of 12 cases of acute mastoiditis or cholesteatoma operated upon between 1978–1987. In these cases the ELS was coincidentally exposed while removing inflamed air cells during mastoidectomy.

Below are the criteria used in classification of the characteristics of the sac.

Position

We followed a slightly modified version of Arenberg et al.'s 3-grade method of classification [8]; our versions of the type I, II, and III categories are illustrated in Figure 11.1. In type I, the ELS is located along Donaldson's line, an imaginary continuation line drawn along the axis of the lateral semicircular canal (LSC). In type III the sac is located far more inferiorly to the posterior semicircular canal (PSC) and close to the jugular bulb; type II is intermediate to type I and III (Figs. 11.1, 11.2).

Size

The ELSs were categorized into 3 groups with regard to size: large, intermediate, and small. "Large" indicates that the length of the sac was more than 6 mm and the width greater than 4 mm; "intermediate" indicates lengths of between 3 mm–6 mm and widths of between 2 mm–4 mm; "small" indicates lengths of under 3 mm and widths of under 2 mm. The sac dimensions were estimated through use of a pick with a tip length of 3 mm.

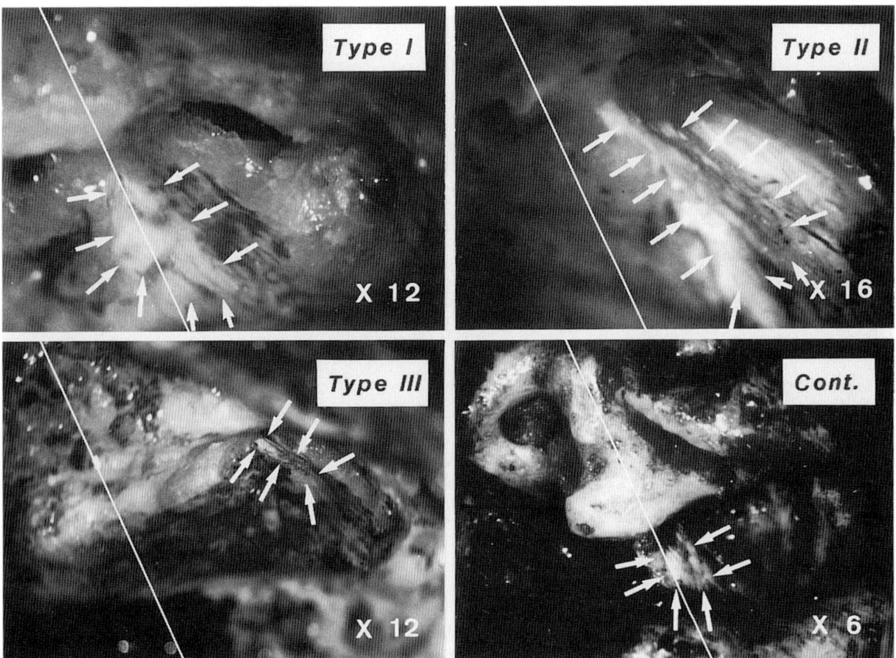

Fig. 11.2. Anatomical classification of the endolymphatic sac position, *type I*, *II*, and *III*, during drainage surgery. A control case with acute mastoiditis displaying type I position. *White lines* indicate the imaginary continuation line drawn along the axis of the lateral semicircular canal (Donaldson's line). *Arrows* indicate the area of the endolymphatic sac

Color

The surface color of the ELS was judged by comparison with the exposed surrounding dura and categorized into 3 grades: red, intermediate, and white. "Red" indicates sacs redder than the surrounding dura, "intermediate" indicates sacs of the same color as the dura, and "white" indicates sacs lighter than the dura.

Vascularity

The vascularity of the ELS was judged from the degree of visible surface capillarization and categorized into 3 groups: fair, intermediate, and poor. "Fair" indicates the presence of a network of 6 capillaries or more; "intermediate" indicates a network of from 3–5 capillaries; "poor" indicates a network of 2 or less capillaries (Fig. 11.3).

Student *t*-tests were used to determine the statistical difference between the Ménière's group and the non-Ménière's group. The correlation between the 4 characteristics was determined through use of chi-squared tests.

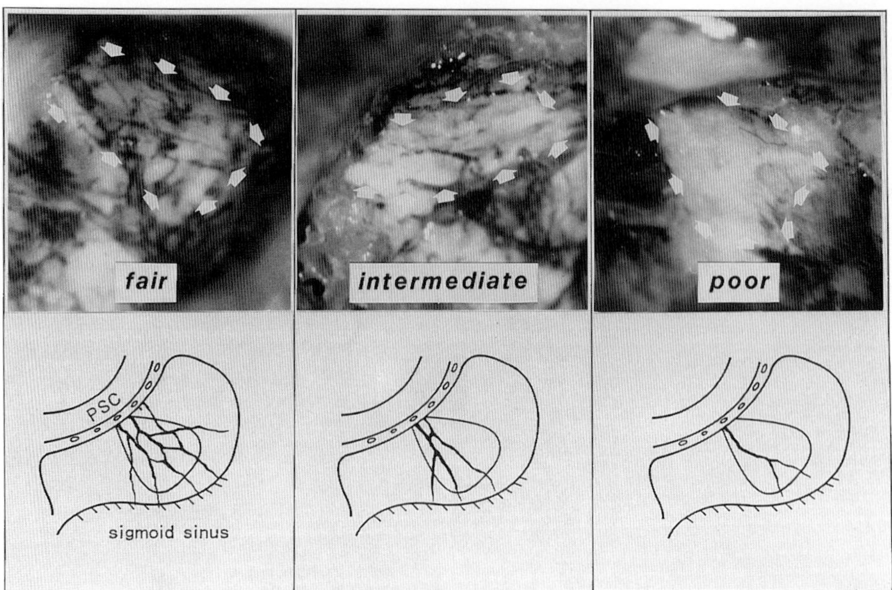

Fig. 11.3. Classification of the ELS vascularity: *fair*, *intermediate* and *poor*. *Arrows* indicate the area of the endolymphatic sac. *PSC*, posterior semicircular canal

Results

The pathoanatomical findings with regard to ELS position, size, color, and vascularity are summarized for both groups in Table 11.1. The details of the findings are as follows.

Position

Among the 46 Ménière's cases there was 1 with type I case (2%), 20 with type II cases (44%), and 25 with type III cases (54%). The Ménière's disease group had a much lower incidence of type I cases and a much higher incidence of type III cases than the control group. Specifically, over half of the Ménière's cases had sacs located inferiorly and anteriorly to the PSC, very close to the jugular bulb. There was, therefore, a significant difference between the Ménière's group and the control group ($P < 0.01$).

Size

The 46 Ménière's cases included 11 cases with large sacs (24%), 19 cases with intermediate-sized sacs (41%), and 16 cases with small sacs (35%). In 3 of the 46 cases the ELSs were not identified during surgery; since this was probably due to the sacs being too small to be noticed, and were counted among the 16 small-sized cases.

Table 11.1. Pathoanatomical findings of the endolymphatic sacs

	Ménière's Disease (46 cases)	Non-Ménière's Disease (12 cases)
Position		
Type I	1 (2%)	5 (42%)
Type II	20 (44%)	6 (50%)
Type III	25 (54%)	1 (8%)
Size		
Large	11 (24%)	5 (42%)
Intermediate	19 (41%)	7 (58%)
Small	16 (35%)	0 (0%)
Color		
Red	1 (2%)	0 (0%)
Intermediate	9 (20%)	8 (67%)
White	36 (78%)	4 (33%)
Vascularity		
Fair	7 (15%)	2 (17%)
Intermediate	15 (33%)	6 (50%)
Poor	24 (52%)	4 (33%)

Although there was a tendency for ELSs in Ménière's disease to be smaller than in non-Ménière's disease, no significant difference was found between the Ménière's group and the control group.

Color

Of the 46 Ménière's cases only 1 (2%) had a red ELS. Nine cases (20%) were intermediate and 36 cases (78%) were white. Although the sac is composed of whitish fibrous tissue even in normal subjects, the Ménière's group had a significantly higher incidence of white coloration than did the control group ($P < 0.01$).

Vascularity

Of the 46 Ménière's cases, 7 (15%) were fair in vascularity, 15 (33%) were intermediate, and 24 (52%) were poor. The incidence of poor vascularity was higher in the Ménière's group than in the control group, but the difference was not significant.

Application of the chi-squared test to the above 4 characteristics revealed a strong correlation between position and size ($P > 0.99$), and between color and vascularity ($P > 0.99$). No significant correlation was found between position and color, position and vascularity, size and color, or size and vascularity.

Discussion

A common finding in the numerous anatomical and radiological studies of the ELS [2–8, 10, 11, 13] has been the great variability in form and position of this structure. Our study investigated the position, size, color and vascularity of the ELS in

Ménière's disease, and attempted to determine the diagnostic significance of these characteristics through statistical evaluation and through comparison with the same characteristics in sacs without Ménière's disease.

The comparisons revealed significant differences only in position and color, indicating that these characteristics are more important in the evaluation of Ménière's disease than size and vascularity. In our study, more than half of the 46 cases of Ménière's disease were of type III classification with regard to ELS position, in which the sacs are located inferiorly and anteriorly to the PSC, close to the jugular bulb. The surface color appeared white in 78% of the cases, far higher than the 33% figure recorded for non-Ménière's cases.

The ELS size has been reported to be rather small in Ménière's disease [2, 6], but no significant difference in sac size were found between the Ménière's and the non-Ménière's disease groups. This result indicates that a small sac size is not a feature strongly characteristic of this condition. As pointed out in a study by Freiberg et al. [12], even normal subjects sometimes display sacs of rudimentary dimensions. In his histological examination of extraosseous portions of 29 normal ELSs, he recorded 2 (7%) in which no ELS epithelium whatsoever was found, and in the remaining 27 specimens, surface areas ranged from 2.1 mm^2–35.9 mm^2, an almost 17-fold differential.

Nevertheless, a definite tendency toward smaller-sized ELSs was seen in our study. This tends to support the findings of Shambaugh [2] and House [6], who noted the diversity in size and location of the extraosseous ELS in Ménière's disease. Shambaugh [2] reported 4 out of 28 cases of Ménière's disease (14%) in which the ELS was completely unidentifiable, and House [6] observed that this structure is rudimentary in about 10% of Ménière's disease cases. In the present study 3 out of 46 cases (6%) were encountered in which the sac could not be identified.

The difference in vascularity between the Ménière's disease group and the control group was not found to be significant. There was, nevertheless, a higher incidence of poor vascularity in Ménière's disease than for the control group (53% vs. 33%), and the possibility does exist that this difference has some bearing on the nature of the disease [2].

Several investigators have noted the high incidence of deficient radiologic reproduction of the VA in patients with Ménière's disease [3, 4, 10]. This finding decided Arenberg et al. [11] to recommend surgery of the endolymphatic sac only on patients in whom tomography has shown the VA to be open. A study of 25 temporal bones from Ménière's disease cases, using the graphic reconstruction method, showed that diminutions of the width of the endolymphatic duct do indeed exist [13]. Nevertheless, it must be remembered that poor visibility of the aqueduct in tomography can also result from technical limitations of the radiogram, and from the curvilinear course of the aqueduct itself in poor or non-pneumatized pyramids.

The reasons for the great variations in its position, size, color and vascularity of the ELS are still unknown, but several possibilities exist related to certain developmental and structural features of the sac. During fetal life, the ELS protrudes posteriorly from the otic capsule. It continues to grow throughout infancy and childhood, and at adulthood is 3 times larger than at birth [1, 2, 14]. The sac, as the only portion of the membranous labyrinth to protrude outside of the otic capsule, may be subject during growth to more frequent contact with viruses and other foreign enemies than other parts of the inner ear, increasing the likelihood of infection and a subsequent deterioration of sac development and function. Furthermore, the capillaries of the ELS are unique in the inner ear, possessing numerous micropores and fenestrations in the endothelial walls [15]. This structural characteristic may also serve to increase the possibility of infection by foreign agents during the developmental period of the sac, resulting in a wide range of sizes and positions in adult ELSs. It is conceivable that this, in turn, could lead to malfunctions related to the later development of endolymphatic hydrops.

Summary

This study attempts to clarify the nature of several of the irregular characteristics of the endolymphatic sac in Ménière's disease. Photographs were taken of the sac in 46 patients with Ménière's disease during endolymphatic sac drainage surgery, and classified into 3 grades with regard to position, size, color and vascularity. A comparison was then made with 12 photographs of the sacs of patients with acute mastoiditis or cholesteatoma. The patients with Ménière's disease were found to have endolymphatic sacs located inferior and more anteriorly to the posterior semicircular canal, very close to the jugular bulb ($P < 0.01$). The sacs were also smaller in size, whiter in surface color ($P < 0.01$) and of less vascularity than those of the patients with non-Ménière's disease. In addition, the chi-squared test revealed significant correlation between the position and size of the sac ($P > 0.99$), and its color and vascularity ($P > 0.99$).

References

1. Anson BJ (1965) The endolymphatic and perilymphatic aqueducts of the human ear: Developmental and adult anatomy of their parietes and contents in relation to otological surgery. Acta Otolaryngol (Stockh) 59: 140–153
2. Shambaugh GE Jr (1966) Surgery of endolymphatic sac. Arch Otolaryngol 83: 305–315
3. Clemis JD, Valvassori GE (1968) Recent radiographic and clinical observations on the vestibular aqueduct. Otolaryngol Clin North Am 10: 339–346
4. Stahle J, Wilbrand H (1974) The vestibular aqueduct in patients with Ménière's disease: A tomographic and clinical investigation. Acta Otolaryngol (Stockh) 78: 36–48
5. Wilbrand HF, Stahle J (1981) Temporal bone in patients with Ménière's disease. In: Vosteen K-H, Schuknecht HF, Pfaltz CR, Wersäll J, Kimura RS, Morgenstern C, Juhn SK (eds) Ménière's disease: Pathogenesis, diagnosis and treatment. Georg Thieme, New York, pp 141–147
6. House WF (1975) Ménière's disease: Management and theory. Otolaryngol Clin North Am 8: 515–535
7. Shambaugh GE Jr, Clemis JD, Arenberg IK (1969) Endolymphatic duct and sac in Ménière's disease. I. Surgical and histopathologic observations. Arch Otolaryngol 89: 816–825
8. Arenberg IK, Rask-Andersen H, Wilbrand H, Stahle J (1977) The surgical anatomy of the endolymphatic sac. Arch Otolaryngol 103: 1–11

9. Kitahara M, Kitajima K, Yazawa Y, Uchida K (1987) Endolymphatic sac surgery for Ménière's disease—17 years experience with the Kitahara sac operation. Am J Otol 8:283–286
10. Kitahara M (1981) Radiological examination. In: Kitahara M (ed) Ménière's disease. Fundamental and clinical observations (in Japanese). Shiga University of Medical Science, Otsu, pp 68–73
11. Arenberg IK, Maroviz WF, Shambaugh GE Jr (1970) The role of the endolymphatic sac in the pathogenesis of endolymphatic hydrops in man. Acta Otolaryngol [Suppl] (Stockh) 275:1–49
12. Freiberg U, Jansson B, Rask-Andersen H, Bagger-Sjoback D (1988) Variations in surgical anatomy of the endolymphatic sac. Otolaryngol Head Neck Surg 114:389–394
13. Ikeda M, Sando I (1984) Endolymphatic duct and sac in patients with Ménière's disease. A temporal bone histopathological study. Ann Otol Rhinol Laryngol 93:540–546
14. Langman J (1963) Ear. In: Langman J (ed) Medical embryology: Human development—normal and abnormal. Williams and Wilkins, Baltimore, pp 293–302
15. Lundquist P-G (1976) Aspects of endolymphatic sac morphology and function. Arch Otorhinolaryngol 212:231–240

CHAPTER 12

Labyrinthine Anomaly and Endolymphatic Hydrops

Haruo Saito, Taizo Takeda, Seiji Kishimoto, and Mutsuhiro Furuta

Goin et al. [1] operated on 16 ears with Mondini's anomaly and obtained satisfactory hearing improvement in 4 of them. Sadé and Yaniv [2] reported on vertigo which started in childhood and suggested that some of the hearing loss with vertigo in children was due to Ménière's disease. Recently, Levenson et al. [3] proposed the existence of the large vestibular aqueduct syndrome in children who have downward fluctuating hearing losses.

These reports suggest that some cases of Ménière's disease have pathogenetic factors starting from early childhood. Early detection of such cases would save these patients from progressive deterioration of their hearing.

The purpose of this study was to determine whether or not there was a correlation between hypoplasty of the labyrinth and endolymphatic hydrops.

Materials and Methods

Twenty-four temporal bones acquired from infants with various congenital anomalies were studied by light microscopy. The ages of the infants ranged from day 0 to 3 months. The specimens were removed at autopsy, fixed, decalcified, embedded in celloidin, and cut horizontally into 20-μm sections. Every 10th section was stained with hematoxylin and eosin.

A search was made for presence of endolymphatic hydrops (EH) in one or more cochlear turns. The grade of EH present was categorized as slight, moderate, or profound, according to the criteria of Paparella et al. [4].

Twenty-four temporal bones without any pathology that was likely produce EH, such as otitis media, served as the controls.

Data were analyzed using Fischer's direct probability test, and $P < 0.05$ was considered significant.

Temporal Bone Histopathological Findings

Endolymphatic hydrops: Of the 24 temporal bones from infants with anomalies, 16 (67%) had EH, whereas it appeared in only 4 of the 24 normal adult temporal bones (17%). The incidence was significantly higher in the congenital anomaly

Table 12.1. Endolymphatic hydrops—grade and distribution

Cochlear turn	Apical lower	upper	Middle lower	upper	Basal lower
Profound	1	0	1	1	1
Moderate	9	4	0	0	0
Slight	0	4	5	3	1
Normal	7	12	18	20	22
Total	[a]17	[b]20	24	24	24

[a] 7 Short cochleae
[b] 4 Short cochleae

group ($P < 0.01$). The grade of EH in the congenital anomaly group was profound in 2 cases, moderate in 12, and slight in 2. EH was found to be more frequent and more severe in the apical turn of the cochlea (Table 1 and Fig. 12.1). Saccular and utricular hydrops was observed in only 4 ears. Saccular hydrops was observed in 2 inner ears in which the cochlear duct was profoundly hydropic. In the other 2 ears, utricular hydrops was slight in both the cochlear duct and the saccule.

Possible etiological factors were studied and analyzed in the 24 ears of the congenital anomaly group.

Hypoplasty of the cochlea: A cochlea with less than two turns was classified as a short cochlea. Six out of 7 (86%) short cochleae and 10 out of 17 (59%) normal length cochleae had EH (P = N.S.).

Wide vestibular aqueduct: fourteen out of 17 (82%) labyrinths with wide vestibular aqueducts had EH, while 2 out of 7 (29%) labyrinths with normal width vestibular aqueducts had EH ($P < 0.05$) (Fig. 12.2).

Foldings and flattened epithelium of the rugous portion of the endolymphatic sac: on the inner surface, foldings were observed in all ears. The lining of the rugous portion of each temporal bone was of cuboidal epithelium, and no flattening of the epithelium was observed in the specimens from the congenital anomaly group.

Silent otitis: The presence of inflammatory cells in the middle ear was also investigated because of the possibility that otitis media could be a causative factor of the EH. Three of the 24 (12%) cases studied in the EH group had inflammatory cells in the middle ear, whereas 1 of the 6 (17%) non-EH cases had inflammatory cells (P = N.S.).

Discussion

Schuknecht and Gulya [5] classified EH into symptomatic and asymptomatic groups, and subdivided them further into embryonic, acquired, and idiopathic groups.

The cases in this report coincide with the asymptomatic embryonic form of Schuknecht and Gulya.

In the present series of temporal bones from infants with congenital anomalies, EH was observed in 67% (16/24) of the cases, while in the controls the incidence

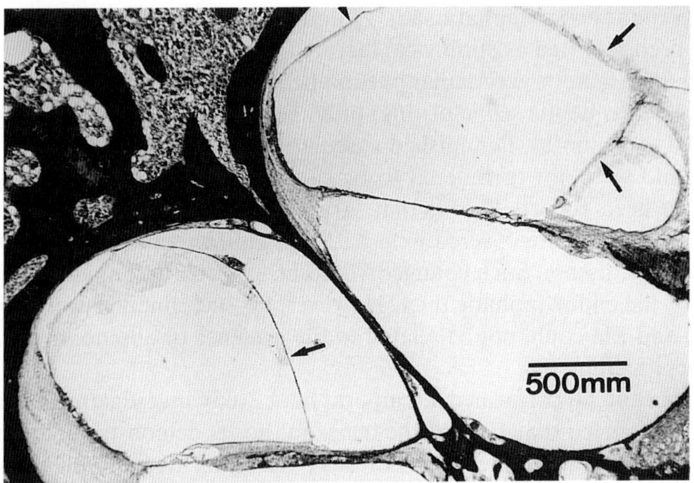

Fig. 12.1. Endolymphatic hydrops in an infant with congenital anomalies. Distention is more severe in the apical turn

was 17% (4/24) ($P < 0.01$). The incidence of EH in the controls in this study was close to the reported incidence of 16% of EH in the apical turn of the normal cochlea [6]. We investigated infants with congenital anomalies to search for possible dysfunction of the endolymphatic fluid excretion and absorption system.

A short cochlea and/or a wide vestibular aqueduct were observed in 79% of the temporal bones in the congenital anomaly group. These findings are recognized as manifestations of labyrinthine hypoplasia. The grade of EH observed in the present series was milder than that reported in adult cases with Ménière's disease. It is possible that the would have progressed with time, if the subjects had lived longer; there would be patients with immature labyrinths which would range between the congenital hypoplasty seen in our series and the fully developed normal labyrinth. The condition of patients with such labyrinths would change with time from asymptomatic to symptomatic due to the gradual accumulation of endolymphatic fluid. Such patients probably represent a part of the symptomatic idiopathic form of EH (Ménière's disease).

In studies of temporal bones acquired from adult patients with Ménière's disease, perisacular fibrosis [7–9], diminished perisacular pneumatization [10, 11], hypo-

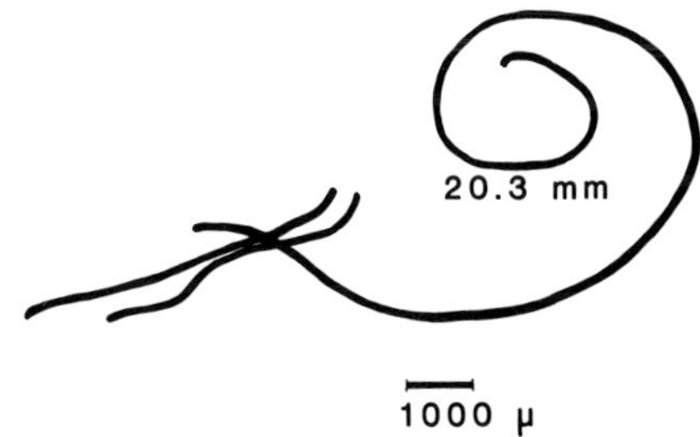

Fig. 12.2. Diagram of the wide vestibular aqueduct in an infant with congenital anomalies

vascularity of the endolymphatic sac [12], and shortening of the vestibular aqueduct [13] have been reported as etiological factors.

Among these factors, perisacular pneumatization and the length of the vestibular aqueduct lie outside the scope of this study, because the ages of our cases ranged from day 0 to 3 months. Diminished vascularity and perisacular fibrosis were not observed and were not considered to be causative factors for EH in this group. There have been reports [7, 14] that large areas of the rugous portion of the endolymphatic sac were covered with flattened epithelium in some adult patients with Ménière's disease. Such changes would be expected to impair the absorptive function of the endolymphatic duct. However, no such findings were observed in our series and EH could not be related to the presence or absence of foldings and flattened epithelium.

Paparella et al. [4] performed a temporal bone study investigating EH and otitis media, and reported that 13% of the temporal bones demonstrated both EH and otitis media. Temporal bones with both EH and otitis media in the present series amounted to 3 out of 24 (12%). This figure is not larger than the incidence in Paparella's report, and the EH showed no relationship to otitis media in the congenital anomaly group.

Since the purpose of this study was to reveal abnormal findings which could be detected by clinical diagnostic methods, the vestibular aqueduct, rather than the endolymphatic duct, was studied. Levenson et al. [3] have recently reported clinical cases in children with downward fluctuating progressive sensorineural hearing loss whose symptoms were thought to be related to the isolated enlargement of the vestibular aqueduct, identified by high-resolution CT.

Our study showed a close correlation between EH and a wide vestibular aqueduct. There might be more children of this type in whom the problem could be detected by careful investigation before the sensorineural hearing loss becomes symptomatic.

Summary

Previous clinical and histopathological evidence has suggested that some cases of Ménière's disease may be congenital. The present study investigated the incidence of EH in temporal bones acquired from infants with congenital anomalies. Serially sectioned temporal bones were studied by light microscopy. EH was significantly more frequent in 24 temporal bones from infants with congenital anomalies than in 24 temporal bones from normal adults ($P < 0.01$). Many of the ears with EH had a wide vestibular aqueduct ($P < 0.05$).

References

1. Goin DW, Rasband RW, Mischke RE, Weaver M (1984) Endolymphatic sac surgery in Mondini's dysplasia: a report of 16 cases. Laryngoscope 94:343–347
2. Sadé J, Yaniv E (1984) Ménière's disease in infants. Acta Otolaryngol (Stockh) 97: 33–37

3. Levenson MJ, Simon C, Jacobs M, Edelstein DR (1989) The large vestibular aqueduct syndrome in children. Arch Otolaryngol Head Neck Surg 115: 54–58
4. Paparella MM, Goycoolea MV, Meyerhoff WF (1979) Endolymphatic hydrops and otitis media. Laryngoscope 89: 43–54
5. Schuknecht HF, Gulya AJ (1983) Endolymphatic hydrops; An overview and classification. Ann Otol Rhinol Laryngol 92 (Suppl 106): 1–20
6. Yamashita T, Schuknecht HF (1982) Apical endolymphatic hydrops. Arch Otolaryngol 108: 463–466
7. Saito H, Kitahara M, Yazawa Y, Matsumoto M (1977) Histopathologic findings in surgical specimens of endolymphatic sac in Ménière's disease. Acta Otolaryngol (Stockh) 83: 465–469
8. Schindler RA (1980) The ultrastructure of the endolymphatic sac in man. Laryngoscope 90 (Suppl 21): 1–39
9. Yazawa Y, Kitahara M (1981) Electron microscopic studies of the endolymphatic sac in Ménière's disease. ORL J Otorhinolaryngol Relat Spec 43: 121–130
10. Stahle J, Wilbrand H (1974) The vestibular aqueduct in patients with Ménière's disease. A tomographic and clinical investigation. Acta Otolaryngol (Stockh) 78: 36–48
11. Sando I, Ikeda M (1985) Histopathological studies in Ménière's disease: Pneumatization and thickness of the petrous bone. Ann Otol Rhinol Laryngol 94 (Suppl 188): 2–5
12. Ikeda M, Sando I (1985) Vascularity of endolymphatic sac in Ménière's disease. A histopathological study. Ann Otol Rhinol Laryngol 94 (Suppl 118): 6–10
13. Rizvi SS, Smith LE (1981) Idiopathic endolymphatic hydrops and vestibular aqueduct. Ann Otol Rhinol Laryngol 90: 77–79
14. Shambaugh GE Jr, Clemis JD, Arenberg IK (1969) The endolymphatic sac and duct in Ménière's disease. I.Surgical and histological observations. Arch Otolaryngol 89: 816–825

CHAPTER 13

An Anatomical Study on Cadavers with a History of Dizziness: Temporal Bone and Some Arteries, Nerve Roots, and Nuclei Related to the Internal Ear

Osamu Tanaka, Haruo Shinohara, and Hiroki Otani

Ménière's disease is characterized by progressive endolymphatic hydrops (EH) of the pars inferior, resulting in the impairment of cochlear and vestibular functions. EH may also occur in syphilitic labyrinthitis [1], delayed endolymphatic hydrops [2–6], petrositis [7], suppurative labyrinthitis [8], congenital deafness [9], and otitis media [10, 11]. Although the cause of EH is unknown, it is widely believed that overaccumulation of endolymph is due either to oversecretion from the stria vascularis or malabsorption through the wall of the endolymphatic duct. At present, there is no morphological evidence related to the pathogenesis of EH.

The aim of the present study was to investigate the relation of the history of vertigo or dizziness with the postmortem anatomical findings in some arteries, nerve roots and nuclei related to the internal ear and in the temporal bones.

Materials and Method

Twenty-one cadavers, 11 men and 10 women, ranging from 59–88 years of age (mean age: 81 years) were included in the present study. In 16 cases there was a history of dizziness, while the remaining 5, without such history, served as the control group. A history of the patient's vestibulocochlear disturbances, obtained by a questionnaire to the attending nurses, provided the basis for the selection of the cadavers. Since the history of dizziness or vertigo was thus obtained from someone other than the patients, the accuracy of the details in not certain. Based on their past histories, most cases had arteriosclerosis, hypertension and heart disease. The cadavers were fixed by perfusion with 10% formalin through the femoral artery. After the brains were removed by dissection, the bodies and brains were separately immersed in the same fixative for more than 6 months.

Arteries, Nerve Roots, and Nuclei Related to the Internal Ear

In this part of the study, the brains from 13 cases were examined, 9 of which had a history of dizziness. The diameters of some regions of the vertebral and basilar arteries were measured by slide calipers. The histology of the VIIIth cranial nerve roots was examined by the luxol fast blue staining method. The sections through three vestibular and two cochlear nuclei were stained with Klüver-Barrera's method in order to number degenerating nerve cells in each nucleus at the level of the abducens nerve nuclei. The degree of stenosis of arteries, degenerating nerve cell ratios in the nuclei, and demyelination of the nerves, were analyzed statistically.

Temporal Bone

Twenty-nine temporal bone materials from 17 cases were obtained with the bone plug method using an oscillating (Stryker) bone plug saw. Of these, 13 cases had a history of vertigo. After decalcification, the specimens were dehydrated in a series of ethyl alcohols and embedded in celloidin. Horizontal sections (20 μm) of the temporal bone were made and stained with hematoxylin-eosin to be studied with a light microscope. Celloidin was washed out by diethyl ether in some sections that were then embedded in Epon 812. Thin sections were cut with a Reichert-Jung OmU_4 ultramicrotome, and stained with uranyl acetate and lead nitrate to be studied with a JEM 200 CX clectron microscope.

Results

Arteries, Nerve Roots, and Nuclei

Atherosclerosis of the vertebral and basilar arteries of various degrees was found in all cases, and more than 50% stenosis was noted in half of the cases (Fig. 13.1). The VIIIth cranial nerve roots exhibited demyelination in some cases. In the vestibular and cochlear nuclei, non specific degenerative findings of nerve cells were observed, such as chromatolysis or ghost cell with the accumulation of lipofuscin (Fig. 13.2). The ratios of degenerating neurons in the vestibular nucleus are shown in Table 13.1. Three cases (*Numbers 375, 414, 376*), of which one had a history of dizziness, had a high ratio of degenerating nerve cells. There was a significant difference in degenerating nerve cell ratio in the right medial vestibular nuclei in cases with a history of dizziness compared to cases with no such history. The degree of the VIIIth cranial nerve demyelination was associated with the degree of stenosis of the right vertebral artery.

Temporal Bone

The relation between premortem history of dizziness and the extension of Reissner's membrane is shown in Table 13.2. Extension of Reissner's membrane was present in 19 out of 22 cochleae of those with dizziness, and in 3 out of 7 cochleae of the controls (Figs. 3 and 4). In addition, moderate extension of Reissner's membrane was observed in 13 out of 29 cochleae of those with dizziness and one out 7 cochleae of the controls (Fig. 13.4). Moderate extension of Reissner's membrane was present in two turns in the left cochlea of case *Number 510* and right cochlea of case *Number 516*.

Brown-pigmented granules were frequently observed in the stria vascularis and the epithelium of the ampulla. In the apical turn of an 80-year-old cadaver (*Number*

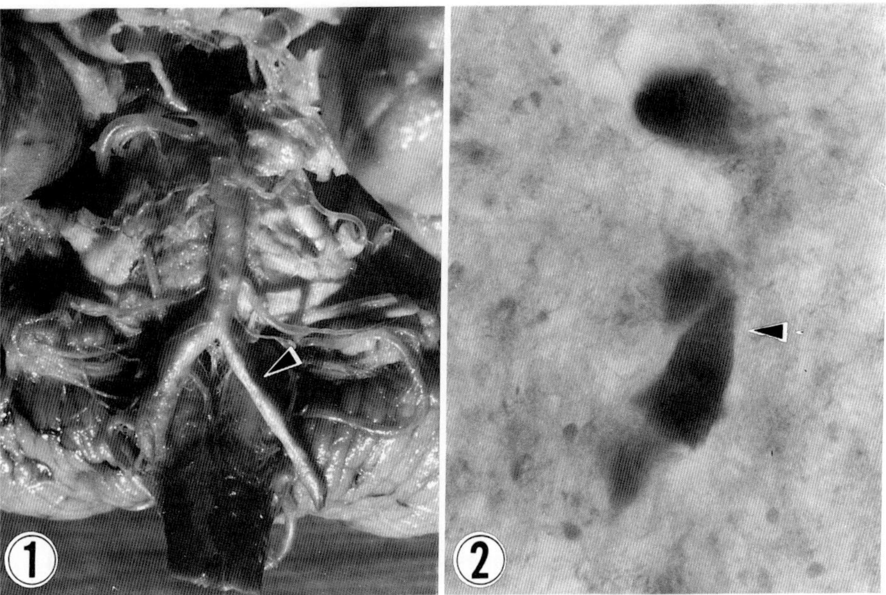

Fig. 13.1. Ventral view of the brain from a cadaver with a history of dizziness. Note that the left vertebral artery is markedly narrowed (*arrowhead*)

Fig. 13.2. A section of the right lateral nucleus of the vestibular nucleus from a cadaver with a history of dizziness, stained by Klüver-Barrera's method The greatest part of the cytoplasm is occupied with lipofuscin (*arrowhead*), X 90

Table 13.1. Ratio of degenerating neurons in the vestibular nucleus

No.	Age (sex)	Vertigo Dizziness	Left Ear sup.	Left Ear lat.	Left Ear med.	Right Ear sup.	Right Ear lat.	Right Ear med.
375	73(F)	–	61.6	65.7	47.3	84.7	61.0	46.7
414	86(F)	–	34.9	34.2	24.2	56.4	52.2	45.2
503	83(F)	–	23.6	20.4	16.7	15.8	18.9	10.5
515	75(M)	–	17.8	21.7	14.6	8.9	14.9	11.6
342	83(M)	+	26.2	21.4	18.0	26.6	25.6	18.0
343	83(M)	+	23.0	19.8	15.7	28.0	21.6	27.6
358	79(M)	+	21.2	23.4	26.1	25.2	18.5	11.1
376	88(F)	+	51.1	69.7	48.4	66.7	49.5	32.1
411	80(M)	+	30.5	24.4	35.3	12.4	25.6	11.2
504	85(M)	+	35.4	35.7	39.8	26.4	32.0	21.9
508	59(M)	+	11.6	51.0	18.4	23.9	43.5	15.1
510	80(F)	+	23.2	38.2	14.2	13.7	40.6	17.7
516	79(F)	+	24.2	23.7	29.5	31.5	22.6	18.7

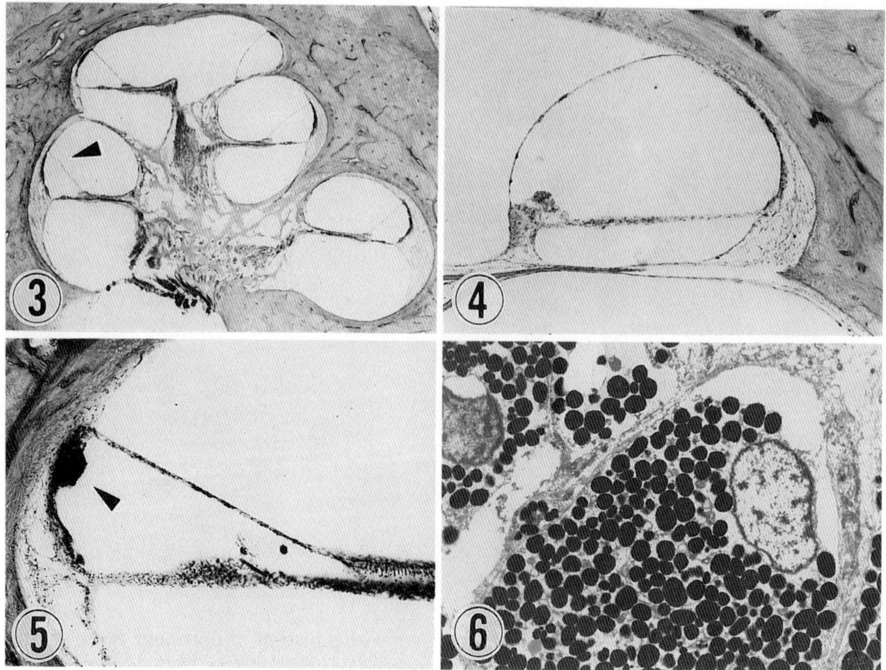

Fig. 13.3. Mid-modiolar section of the left cochlea from a cadaver with a history of dizziness. Reissner's membrane at the apical turn is slightly distended and a fold is present in the middle turn *(arrowhead)*, X 10

Fig. 13.4. Apical turn of the right cochlea from a cadaver with a history of dizziness, showing moderate extension of Reissner's membrane, X 47

Fig. 13.5. Pigmented granule observed in the stria vascularis (*arrowhead*) of the left cochlea from a cadaver with a history of dizziness, X 46

Fig. 13.6. Ultrastructure of the pigmented granule in the epithelium of the ampulla from a cadaver with a history of dizziness. Electron-dense round granules are observed in the cytoplasm, X 2700

411), with a history of sudden episodes of dizziness or vertigo associated with tinnitus, a mass of brown or black pigmentation was observed (Fig. 13.5). These granules were not discolored by treatment with hydrogen peroxide. Electron microscopic study showed that these pigmented granules were clusters of oval electron-dense granules in the cytoplasm of the epithelial cells (Fig. 13.6).

Discussion

One of the approaches of obtaining the temporal bone findings associated with dizziness is described. Degenerating nerve cells were frequently observed in some cases with a history of dizziness; however, the relation between such degenerating

Table 13.2. Distension of Reissner's membrane (From [10])

No.	Age (sex)	Vertigo Dizziness	Left Ear basal	Left Ear middle	Left Ear apical	Right Ear basal	Right Ear middle	Right Ear apical
360	88 M	−	−	+	+	−	−	+
375	73 F	−	−	−	−	−	−	−
414	86 F	−	−	−	−	−	−	+ +
515	75 M	−				−	−	−
363	78 M	+	−	−	+			
364	86 F	+	+	+	+ +	+	+	+ +
376	88 F	+				−	−	+
405	76 F	+	+	+	+ +	−	−	−
411	80 M	+	−	−	+ +	−	−	+ +
463	85 M	+	+	+	+ +	+	+	+
474	87 F	+	+	+	+ +	+	+	+ +
477	89 F	+	−	+	+	−	+	+
478	82 M	+	−	−	−	−	+	+
504	85 M	+	+	+	+ +			
508	59 M	+	−	−	−	+	+	+
510	80 F	+	+ +	+ +	+			
516	79 F	+	+	+	+ +	+	+ +	+ +

M, male; F, female; +, slight; + +, moderate

nerve cells and the pathological findings in the corresponding arteries could not be determined in the present study.

Extension of Reissner's membrane was more frequently observed in the cochleae of patients with a history of dizziness. The extension at the apical turn was observed in 19 out of 22 cochleae from these cases but only in 3 out of 7 cochleae in the control group. However, such apical hydrops are believed to be of no pathological or functional significance [12, 13]. It is noteworthy that moderate extension of Reissner's membrane was observed in two turns each of two cochleae from cases with a history of dizziness. This is in accord with the generally accepted notion that cochlear hydrops is the common pathological finding in the temporal bones with Ménière's disease [14].

Some investigators have reported brown pigmentation [15–18] and hyalinization of perisaccular tissue [16, 19], and intraluminal eosinophilic precipitate [20] of the endolymphatic sac in temporal bones from individuals with Ménière's disease. In the present study, many pigmented granules were found in the stria vascularis and epithelium of the ampulla. Our impression is that these granules appear more frequently in patients with a history of dizziness. Huge masses were observed by electron microscopy in the endothelial cells of the stria vascularis in specimens of Ménière's disease [21]. It is possible that the presence of such granules may stimulate the secretion of endolymph from the stria vascularis, resulting in cochlear hydrops. However, these pigmented granules were observed in almost all the cases examined, even in the cochleae of the control group. Since the number of our cases is small, we are thereby restricted in evaluating the relationship between pigmented granules and the history of vertigo, and more cases have to be studied before drawing any conclusions. The authors are fully aware of the limitations of this temporal bone study, based as it is on retrospective information concerning the history of dizziness.

We studied the temporal bones and some tissues related to the function of the inner ear from cadavers with a past history of dizziness, in which endolymphatic hydrops resembling the common pathological finding of Ménière's disease was frequently observed. The approach we used in the present study may be helpful in studying the pathological changes that take place in well-documented cases of Ménière's disease.

References

1. Karmody C, Schuknecht HF (1966) Deafness in congenital syphilis. Arch Otolaryngol 83:18–27
2. Wolfson R, Leiberman A (1975) Unilateral deafness with subsequent vertigo. Laryngoscope 85:1752–1766
3. Nadol J, Weiss A, Parker S (1975) Vertigo of delayed onset after sudden deafness with subsequent vertigo. Laryngoscope 84:841–846
4. Schuknecht HF (1978) Delayed endolymphatic hydrops. Ann Otol Rhinol Laryngol 87:743–748
5. Kamei T (1978) Delayed vertigo. In: Hood JD (ed) Vestibular mechanisms in health and disease. Academic, New York, pp 369–374
6. LeLiever WC, Barber HO (1980) Delayed endolymphatic hydrops. J Otolaryngol 9: 375–380
7. Allam AF, Schuknecht (1968) Pathology of petrositis. Laryngoscope 78:1813–1832
8. Paparella MM, Sugiura S (1967) The pathology of suppurative labyrinthitis. Ann Otol Rhinol Laryngol 76:554–586
9. Cohn AM, Beal DD, Kohut RI (1968) Inner ear pathology in unilateral congenital deafness. Ann Otol Rhinol Laryngol 77:43–53
10. Paparella MM, Goycoolea MV, Meyerhoff WL (1979) Endolymphatic hydrops and otitis media. Laryngoscope 89:43–54
11. Saito H, Kitahara M, Kitajima K, Takeda T, Yazawa Y, Matsubara H, Kitano H (1981) Distended Reissner's membrane and otitis media (in Japanese). Pract Otol (Kyoto) 74 (Suppl 5):2413–2417
12. Ishii T (1977) Endolymphatic hydrops in the apical turn (in Japanese). Pract Otol (Kyoto) 70 (Suppl 5):1578–1761
13. Yamashita T, Schuknecht HF (1982) Apical endolymphatic hydrops. Arch Otolaryngol 108:463–467
14. Paparella MM (1985) The cause (multifactorial inheritance) and pathogenesis (endolymphatic malabsorption) of Ménière's disease and its symptoms (mechanical and chemical). Acta Otolaryngol (Stockh) 99:445–451
15. Altman F, Fowler EP (1943) Histological findings in Ménière's symptom comple. Ann Otol Rhinol Laryngol 52:52–80
16. Sando I, Holinger LD, Balkany T, Wood RP II (1976) Unilateral endolymphatic hydrops and associated abnormalities. Ann Otol Rhinol Laryngol 85:368–376
17. Saito H, Kitahara M, Yazawa Y, Matsumoto M (1977) Histopathologic findings in surgical specimens of the endolymphatic sac in Ménière's disease. Acta Otolaryngol (Stockh) 83:465–469
18. Zechner G, Altman F (1969) Histological studies on the human endolymphatic duct and sac. Practica Oto-rhino-laryngologica 31:65–83
19. Gussen R. (1974) Ménière's syndrome: Compensatory collateral venous drainage with endolymphatic sac fibrosis. Arch Otolaryngol 99:414–418
20. Ikeda M, Sando I (1984) Endolymphatic duct and sac in patients with Ménière's disease. A temporal bone histopathologic study. Ann Otol Rhinol Laryngol 93:540–546
21. Kimura RS, Schuknecht HF (1970) The ultrastructure of the human stria vascularis. Part II. Acta Otolaryngol (Stockh) 70:301–318

Part III. Symptomatology and Diagnosis of Ménière's Disease

CHAPTER 14

A Statistical Study on Patients with Ménière's Disease Visiting Our Clinic During the Past 10 Years

Yoshiro Wada, Isao Koh, Katsuya Akioka, Nobuya Fujita, Takashi Matsunaga, and Hisami Iwasaki

The etiology of Ménière's disease remains unknown despite many extensive studies [1, 2]. For this reason, the term Ménière's disease is rather widely defined, and there is still no general agreement for diagnosis and treatment [3–5]. To elucidate this problem, we have observed patients with Ménière's disease in the Vertigo Clinic of our hospital for 10 years. In this study, we report several clinical characteristics of Ménière's disease and discuss them in comparison with other reports in the literature.

Materials and Methods

One hundred and eighty patients with confirmed Ménière's disease, seen in our clinic during the period from 1977 to 1986, were investigated. The criteria for establishing the diagnosis were taken from the Ménière's Disease Research Committee of Japan, 1974. Detailed medical histories were taken from all patients, and each was subjected to routine equilibrium function tests on the first visit.

Results

Patient Analysis

The incidence of Ménière's disease for all vertigo-related diseases was 8%, and for all diseases was 0.28% in our clinic. The annual number of patients with Ménière's disease during our study was irregular (Fig. 14.1). The total number of females (109) was about one and a half times as many as that of males (71).

The age distribution peaked in the age group of 50–59 years for males, and for females at 40–49 years (Fig.14.2). The mean age for males (45.3 years) was similar to that for females (47.4 years). Figure 14.3 shows the proportion of patients over 60 years old. They were divided into two groups according to the duration of the study, i.e., the first 5 years and the last 5 years. The proportion of both sexes increased with that of females being more than that of males in each period.

In the spring, especially in April and May, the number of patients was slightly higher than that in other seasons (Fig. 14.4).

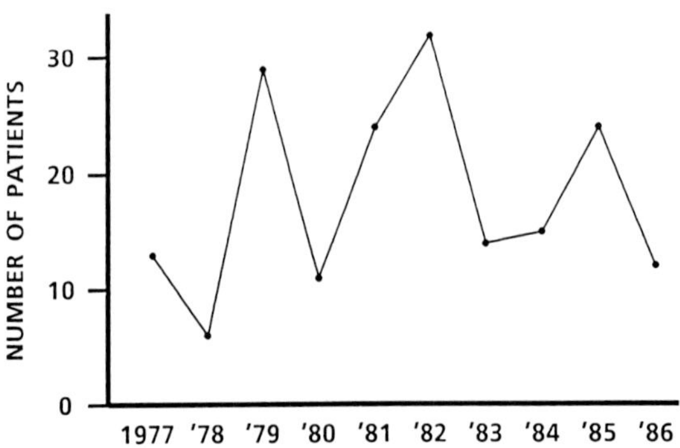

Fig. 14.1. Annual number of patients with Ménière's disease in our clinic during the period from 1977 to 1986

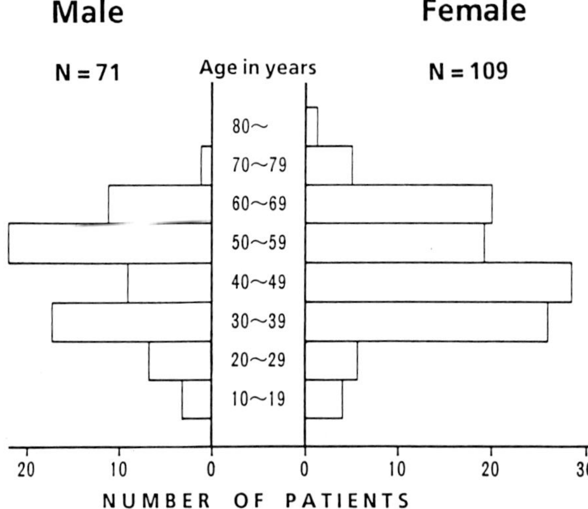

Fig. 14.2. Age distribution of male and female patients with Ménière's disease

Table 14.1. The period from the first vertigo attack until coming to our clinic

Period	Patients
< 1 week	18 (11%)
1 week to 1 month	37 (23%)
1 month to 3 months	20 (13%)
3 months to 1 year	15 (9%)
1 year to 3 years	29 (18%)
3 years to 10 years	29 (18%)
> 10 years	11 (7%)
Total	159 (100%)

Table 14.2. Results of righting reflex tests and deviation tests

Test	Patients
Righting reflex tests	
Normal	60 (59%)
Intermediate	18 (18%)
Abnormal	23 (23%)
Total	101 (100%)
Deviation tests	
Normal	80 (79%)
Intermediate	13 (13%)
Abnormal	8 (8%)
Total	101 (100%)

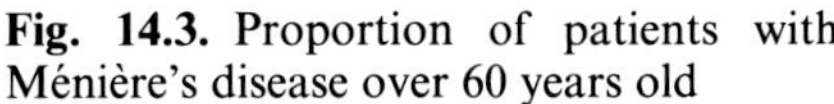

Fig. 14.3. Proportion of patients with Ménière's disease over 60 years old

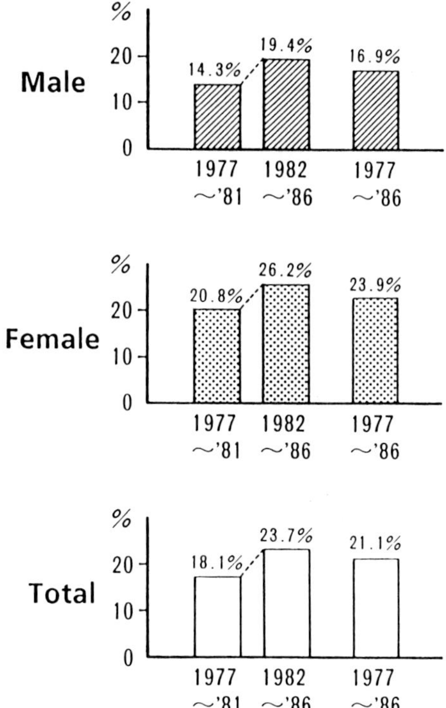

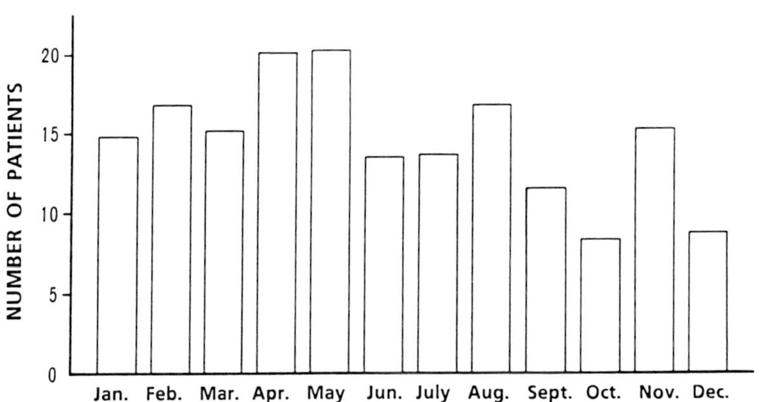

Fig. 14.4. Monthly number of patients with Ménière's disease

The period from the first vertigo attack until presenting at our clinic varied greatly (Table 14.1). One-third of the patients came within one month, whereas a quarter of the patients came more than three years after the onset of vertigo.

Symptoms

On the first visit to our clinic, 52% of the patients presented with vertigo as the chief complaint, while 24% complained of gait disturbance, a more severe symptom than vertigo. Following these vestibular symptoms, cochlear symptoms such as tinnitus (16%) and hearing loss (8%) were also primary symptoms.

With regard to laterality, on the basis of the clinical symptology, 41% of the patients were diagnosed as right side Ménière's disease, 53% were left side, and 6% were bilateral.

On the first attack, patients complained of not only vertigo (76%) but also of nonrotatory dizziness (20%) and other kinds of vestibular symptoms (4%).

Attacks of vertigo were accompanied by other symptoms in addition to hearing loss and tinnitus, such as fullness in the ear (38%), vomiting (28%) and shoulder stiffness (27%).

Results of Routine Equilibrium Function Tests

Righting Reflex Tests and Deviation Tests

Righting reflex evaluation included Romberg's test, Mann's test, and standing on one foot. Deviation evaluation included walking, stepping and writing tests. Judging from all tests collectively, 23% of the patients had abnormalities in righting reflex tests, while 8% revealed abnormalities in deviation tests (Table 14.2).

Nystagmus Tests

We measured the spontaneous, fixation, positional, and positioning nystagmus of the patients. Positional (33%) and positioning (37%) were observed more fre-

Table 14.3. Results of nystagmus tests

Nystagmus test	Patients
Spontaneous nystagmus	
(−)	146 (99%)
(+)	2 (1%)
Total	148 (100%)
Fixation nystagmus	
(−)	133 (89%)
(+)	17 (11%)
Total	150 (100%)
Positional nystagmus	
(−)	87 (67%)
(+)	43 (33%)
Total	130 (100%)
Positioning nystagmus	
(−)	61 (64%)
(+)	35 (37%)
Total	96 (100%)

quently in comparison with spontaneous (1%) and fixation nystagmus (11%) (Table 14.3).

Carolic Testing

During the period of nystagmus following irrigation with 50 ml of water at either 30°C or 44°C for 15 sec we determined the presence of canal paresis (CP) and directional preponderance (DP). Twenty-eight percent of the patients were judged as having CP, 7% had DP and 6% had CP + DP (Table 14.4).

Discussion

There were some differences between the many physicians who reported statistical studies on patients with Ménière's disease [6, 7]. This is not surprising since the features of patients with Ménière's disease differ with the reporting times, the criteria for the diagnosis, the area of hospital (urban vs. rural), the kind of clinic (general vs. specialized), and so on. We will clarify several distinctions between our results and those of others, and discuss the reasons for these differences.

The incidence of Ménière's disease for all diseases in ENT clinics was reported to be from 0.5%–5% [8, 9]. The number of female patients was almost the same as or slightly greater than that of males [10, 11]. However, according to our study, the incidence was 0.28% and the female/male ratio was about 3 : 2. We think the reasons for these differneces are as follows: our hospital is situated in the center of Nara, a suburb of Osaka city. Quite a large number of men living in Nara are employed in Osaka. Generally, when they complain of vertigo, they tend to go to the hospitals in Osaka. Therefore the incidence of Ménière's disease and the number of males were slightly low in our clinic. However, the incidence of Ménière's disease in all vertigo diseases was reported to be about 10% [12, 13] and our data (8%) corresponded with this.

It has been reported that there is no correlation between the attack of Ménière's disease and the season of the year [14]. Our data, however, shows that patients tend to visit our clinic in the spring when sudden changes in temperature may cause the stress which triggers the attack of Ménière's disease.

Table 14.4. Results of Caloric test

Result	Patients
Normal	83 (59%)
CP	39 (28%)
DP	10 (7%)
CP + DP	9 (6%)
Total	141 (100%)

The frequency of bilateral involvement was reported as high as 76% or as low as 9% [15, 16]: in our study it was very low (6%). As it appears to depend upon the length of time patients are kept under observation, we will have to observe them for and carefully monitor the uninvolved ear.

References

1. Gundrum LK (1953) Etiologic analysis of one hundred cases of Ménière's symptom-complex. Arch Otolaryngol 57:123–128
2. Schmidt PH, Brunsting RC, Antvelink JB (1979) Ménière's disease: Etiology and natural history. Acta Otolaryngol (Stockh) 87:410–412
3. Sjöberg A (1964) Clinical experience from the treatment of Ménière's disease. Acta Otolaryngol [Suppl] (Stockh) 192:139–153
4. Pulec JL (1972) Ménière's disease: Results of a two and one half year study of etiology, natural history and results of treatment. Laryngoscope 82:1703–1715
5. Thomsen J, Geisler PB, Jörgensen MB, Rafaelsen OJ, Terkildsen K, Udsen J, Zilstorff K (1974) Ménière's disease; Preliminary report of lithium treatment. Acta Otolaryngol (Stockh) 78:59–64
6. Naito T (1973) Ménière's disease (in Japanese). Pract Otol (Kyoto) 66:1–48
7. Wada Y, Koh I, Akioka K, Fujita N, Matsunaga T, Iwasaki H (1990) A statistical observation of current patients with Ménière's disease in our clinic (in Japanese). Pract Otol (Kyoto) (to be published)
8. Morrison AW (1984) Ménière's disease. In: Dix MR, Hood JD (eds) Vertigo. Wiley, Chichester, pp 133–154
9. Colman BH (1987) Ménière's disease. In: Booth JB (ed) Otology. Butterworths, London, pp 444–464 (Scott-Brown's otolaryngology, vol 3)
10. Permin PM, Poulsen H (1956) Ménière's disease; Follow-up on 371 patients treated in hospital by conservative measures. Acta Otolaryngol (Stockh) 47:219–230
11. Watanabe I (1981) Ménière's disease in males and females. Acta Otolaryngol (Stockh) 91:511–514
12. Mizukoshi K, Kato I, Ishikawa k, Aoyagi M, Watanabe Y, Yamazaki H, Hojo K, Ohno Y (1975) Neurotological studies of Ménière's disease (in Japanese). Pract Otol (Kyoto) 68:1353–1366
13. Matsunaga T, Tagami E, Takimoto K, Okumura S, Yamada S, Naito T (1976) Statistical observation of Ménière's disease (in Japanese). Otolaryngol (Tokyo) 48:65–71
14. Hashimoto M, Tokita T, Miyata H, Hayano Y, Maki T, Maeda M, Kato T (1975) Studies on predisposition to Ménière's disease (in Japanese). Pract Otol (Kyoto) 68: 1379–1388
15. Kitahara M, Matsubara H, Takeda T (1975) Bilateral Ménière's disease (in Japanese). Pract Otol (Kyoto) 68:1389–1394
16. Oosterveld WJ (1979) Ménière's disease: a survey of 408 patients. Acta Otorhinolaryngol Belg 33:428–431

CHAPTER 15

Prediction of Prognosis for Hearing in Ménière's Disease

Kanemasa Mizukoshi, Shin Aso, and Yukio Watanabe

In patients with Ménière's disease, hearing has been known to fluctuate, especially in the early stages. In some cases, even in early stages, however, hearing deteriorates progressively and never recovers. If these cases could be predicted, we could try an intensive treatment in an effort to prevent hearing loss, calling up on both surgical and conservative techniques without delay.

In this paper, the authors will discuss whether or not the glycerol test and/or the electrocochleography (ECochG) could provide information for predicting the prognosis for hearing in Ménière's disease.

Materials and Methods

This study was conducted on 136 cases of Ménière's disease, of which 26 were affected bilaterally. There were 78 females and 58 males. Their ages ranged from 15–77 years with a mean of 48.5 years. For the diagnosis of Ménière's disease, criteria proposed by Ménière's Disease Research Committee were applied [1].

Pure tone audiometry was carried out on all patients. The average hearing threshold was calculated for the frequencies 0.5, 1 and 2 kHz. The glycerol test was applied on 81 cases and the ECochG on 77 cases. For the glycerol test, pure tone audiometry was carried out immediately before and 30, 60, 90, and 120 min after an intravenous injection of 500 ml of 10% glycerol. Improvement of 10 dB or more at 2 or more frequencies was regarded as a positive test result. For the ECochG, the transtympanic method with clicks of 100 dB SPL was used. A test result with larger than 0.37 SP/AP ratio was defined as positive.

These results were analyzed retrospectively in regard to the prognosis of hearing status.

Results

The average hearing threshold at the first visit to our hospital was investigated in relation to the duration of the disease, i.e., the time between the first vertiginous attack and the examination (Table 15.1). Patients with a longer duration of the

Table 15.1. Hearing in relation to duration of illness

Duration of illness (years)	Average hearing threshold (0.5, 1, 2kHz) 0–30 dB	30–60 dB	60–90 dB	Total (cases)
0–1	20	22	8	50
1–2	7	4	4	15
2–3	1	5	2	8
3–4	1	3	3	7
4–5	0	1	2	3
5–	5	11	11	27
Total (cases)	34	46	30	110

disease generally had a more profound hearing loss. No patient listed in Table 15.1 had an average hearing threshold of more than 90 dB.

It was possible for pure tone audiometry to be carried out 1 year after baseline testing in 29 patients, excluding those who underwent endolymphatic sac surgery during this period. Except for the 3 cases who visited our hospital within 1 year after the onset of the first attack, none of the patients showed an improvement in hearing (Table 15.2).

Table 15.3 shows the results of the glycerol test and the ECochG in 14 cases of Ménière's disease whose duration of the disease was less than 1 year. It was possible to perform pure tone audiometry on all of them 1 year after the glycerol test and/or the ECochG. Patients who underwent endolymphatic surgery during the above period are excluded from this Table. In Table 15.3, "unchanged" refers to changes in the average hearing threshold no greater than 5 dB. Of 9 patients with a positive glycerol test, hearing in 3 cases was improved, while in 5 patients with a negative glycerol test, the hearing threshold in 4 cases deteriorated. In other words, hearing improvement was observed only in cases with a positive glycerol test, and hearing in most cases with a negative glycerol test deteriorated. The above tendency differences were not observed from the results of ECochG in cases either with dominant negative SP or normal negative SP.

Table 15.2. Changes in hearing one year after baseline audiometry in relation to the intervals between onset and follow-up

Interval (years)	Hearing one year after baseline audiometry Worse	Improved	Unchanged	Total (cases)
0–1	1	3	9	13
1–2	0	0	6	6
2–3	0	0	0	0
3–4	2	0	0	2
4–5	0	0	0	0
5–	1	0	7	8
Total	4	3	22	29

Table 15.3. Prognostic value of the glycerol test and ECochG in hearing

Results of Gly. and EcochG	Hearing one year after baseline audiometry				Total (cases)
	Worse	Improved	Fluctuating	Unchanged	
Glycerol (+)	1	3	1	4	9
Glycerol (−)	4	0	0	1	5
Enlarged -SP	4	2	1	3	10
Normal -SP	2	1	0	1	4

Discussion

In this study, it was revealed that the hearing of patients whose duration of the disease was less than 1 year could be improved more than 10 dB in 10%, and more than 20 dB in only 3% (1 case) out of 29 cases using conservative treatment. Without exception, the hearing of patients whose duration of the disease was more than 1 year could not be improved. It must be understood that hearing in Ménière's disease is very difficult to maintain or improve with conservative treatment, and that any treatment should preferably carried out at an early stage.

In order to predict the prognosis of hearing in Ménière's disease, the authors carried out the glycerol test and the ECochG for patients at an early stage and monitored their hearing for 1 year. We found that in some patients with a positive glycerol test hearing was improved, while in most patients with a negative glycerol test hearing deteriorated. In general, a positive glycerol test is more frequently detected in early rather than in advanced stages. In our study, a positive glycerol test was observed in 32 (60%) out of 53 cases when the duration of the disease was less than 3 years, while it was observed in only 10 out of 28 cases (35%) when the disease had been present more than 3 years. According to Tonndorf [2], both Reissner's and the basilar membranes are elastic and can be displaced in accordance with their compliance ratio in acute conditions, but Reissner's membrane is found to be overextended in chronic conditions. This hypothesis could explain the above findings.

Patients at an early stage could be classified into 3 groups with regard to the prognosis for hearing.

Patients whose hearing has already deteriorated more than 60 dB at an early stage.

As Enander and Stahle [3] reported, the dominant part of hearing loss develops relatively early in the course of Ménière's disease. As shown in Table 15.1, hearing in 8 out of 50 patients (16%), with a disease duration of less than 1 year, deteriorated between 60–90 dB. They were treated medically or surgically. However, hearing in half of these patients, monitored for 1 year, did not recover even though most showed a positive glycerol test. The above 8 patients were in acute condition and might indeed have had good elasticity of both Reissner's and the basal membranes resulting in positive in a glycerol tests, yet they didn't show good prognosis of hearing despite medical and/or surgical treatment. Therefore, it can be speculated that the critical point between reversible and irreversible hearing is from the range of 60 dB more. A larger number of patients who experienced rapid deterioration of hearing will not be able to recover their hearing even at an early stage.

Patients with a negative glycerol test at an early stage.

Since in most patients with Ménière's disease the hearing deteriorates, it is vital to apply intensive treatment quickly. Though the results of endolymphatic sac surgery are poor in these cases [4, 5], the decision of whether or not to operate must be made immediately.

Patients with a positive glycerol test at an early stage.

The treatment results are not satisfactory although at least hearing does not become worse within 1 year. Surgical and/or medical treatment should be considered in the early stage because Reissner's and the basilar membranes still have some elasticity and can be reversed to an improved condition.

For predicting hearing prognosis the ECochG has little value.

References

1. Watanabe I (1980) Ménière's disease. With special emphasis on epidemiology, diagnosis and prognosis. ORL J Otorhinolaryngol Relat Spec 42:20–45
2. Tonndorf J (1975) Mechanical causes of fluctuant hearing loss. Otolaryngol Clin North Am 8:303–311
3. Enander A, Stahle J (1967) Hearing in Ménière's disease. A study of pure tone audiograms in 334 patients. Acta Otolaryngol (Stockh) 64:543–556
4. Shea JJ (1968) Surgery of the endolymphatic sac. Otolaryngol Clin North Am 1:613–621
5. Sauer RC, Kaemmerle AW, Arenberg IK (1980) The prognostic value of the glycerol test. A review of 60 ears with unidirectional inner ear valve implants. Otolaryngol Clin North Am 13:693–701

CHAPTER 16

A Clinical Study of the Diagnosis of the Endolymphatic Hydrops Aspect of Ménière's Disease

Katsuya Akioka, Nobuya Fujita, Yoshiyuki Kitaoku, and Takashi Matsunaga

Hydrops of the endolymphatic system is the most striking pathologic finding in the inner ear in Ménière's disease. It was discovered simultaneously by Yamakawa [1] and Hallpike and Cairns [2] in 1938 and has subsequently been confirmed by numerous investigations. In our study, the glycerol test, the electrocochleogram (ECochG) and the furosemide tests with caloric stimuli and/or centric & eccentric pendular rotation stimuli were administered to patients with Ménière's disease. The purpose of the study was to diagnose endolymphatic hydrops in these patients in comparison with that in patients with sudden deafness without vertigo.

Materials and Methods

Materials

We studied 92 patients (42 males and 50 females) who were treated in the vertigo clinic in the E.N.T. department of our hospital for 8 years (April, 1981–March, 1989), and who had undergone at least one of the following: the glycerol test, the ECochG and the furosemide tests with caloric stimuli and/or centric & eccentric pendular rotation stimuli. They included 65 patients with confirmed Ménière's disease (71 ears) and 27 patients with suspected Ménière's disease (27 ears). The mean age was 47.4 years (Table 16.1). The control group, patients with sudden deafness without vertigo, consisted of 53 patients, 27 males and 26 females, with a mean age of 46.7 years (Table 16.1).

Methods

First we studied the rate of positive test results for the patients with Ménière's disease in comparison with the group with sudden deafness without vertigo. Second, we compared the rate of positive test results for the patients with confirmed Ménière's disease with the group with suspected Ménière's disease. Third, we studied the rate of positive test results during vertigo attacks and during the vertigo remission stage. Finally we used the test results to diagnose the endolymphatic hydrops aspect of 26 patients with Ménière's disease. These 26 patients had under-

Table 16.1. Patient profile

Disease	Number of cases	Sex		Age		Location of disease		
		Male	Female	Distribution	Mean	Right	Left	Bilateral
Ménière's disease	92	42	50	15 ~ 73	47.4	29	57	6
Sudden deafness without vertigo	53	27	26	13 ~ 74	46.7	18	34	1

gone all the four tests described above. The methods and the criteria used for the tests are as follows:

Glycerol test

A pure tone audiogram was obtained before and 3 hours after administration of 50% glycerin (Amilac; 2.4 ml/kg body weight), using Klockhoff and Lindblom's method [3].

Electrocochleogram

The ECochG was administered extratympanically and with the stimulation of a click sound. Patients who showed a ratio of more than 0.35–SP/AP were considered to react positively.

Furosemide tests

Furosemide test with centric & eccentric pendular rotation stimuli. This test was performed according to Okumura et al.'s method [4]. Furosemide test with caloric stimuli was performed according to Futaki and Kitahara's method [5].

Statistical method

We used the χ^2-test to obtain values with a 5% error rate.

Results

Positive Test Results for Ménière's Disease

Comparison with Sudden Deafness Without Vertigo

We studied Ménière's disease in 92 patients (98 ears) and sudden deafness without vertigo in 53 patients (54 ears) in terms of positive test results (Table 16.2). The rates of positive glycerol test results were 47% for Ménière's disease and 29% for sudden deafness without vertigo. The rates of positive responses on the ECochG were 69% for Ménière's disease and 23% for sudden deafness without vertigo. For the furosemide test with centric & eccentric pendular rotation stimuli, the rates were 32% for Ménière's disease and 0% for sudden deafness without vertigo. These results show that for all three tests, the group with Ménière's disease had significantly higher positive rates. The rates of positive results for the furosemide

Table 16.2. Positive response rates for the tests for Ménière's disease compared with those for sudden deafness without vertigo

Disease	*Glycerol test	*Electrocochleogram	Furosemide tests	
			*Pendular rotation stimuli	Caloric stimuli
Ménière's disease ($n = 98$)	47% (45/95)	69% (33/48)	32% (9/28)	44% (14/32)
Sudden deafness without vertigo ($n = 54$)	29% (13/44)	23% (5/22)	0% (0/11)	20% (2/10)

Numbers in parentheses represent positive cases per total number of cases tested
$*P < 0.05$ (X^2 – test)

test with caloric stimuli were 44% for Ménière's disease and 20% for sudden deafness without vertigo. The rate was thus higher for the group with Ménière's disease, but the value was not significant.

Comparison with Suspected Ménière's Disease

A comparison of the rates for the two groups is shown in Table 16.3. The rates of positive glycerol test results were 51% for confirmed, and 38% for suspected Ménière's disease. The rates of positive responses on the ECochG were 71% for confirmed Ménière's disease and 50% for suspected Ménière's disease. The rates of positive results for the furosemide test with centric & eccentric pendular rotation stimuli were 42% for confirmed and 11% for suspected Ménière's disease. For all three tests, the group with confirmed Ménière's disease showed significantly higher positive rates. The rates of positive results for the furosemide test with caloric stimuli were 39% for confirmed Ménière's disease and 56% for suspected Ménière's disease. The latter group thus showed a significantly higher positive rate.

Table 16.3. Positive response rates for the tests for confirmed Ménière's disease in comparison with those for suspected Ménière's disease

Disease	Glycerol test	Electrocochleogram	Furosemide tests	
			Pendular rotation stimuli	Caloric stimuli
Confirmed Ménière's disease ($n = 71$)	51% (35/69)	71% (27/38)	42% (8/19)	39% (9/23)
Suspected Ménière's disease ($n = 27$)	38% (10/26)	50% (5/10)	11% (1/9)	56% (5/9)

Numbers in parentheses represent the number of positive cases per total number of cases tested

Table 16.4. Positive response rates for the tests for Ménière's disease performed during vertigo attacks in comparison with those performed during the vertigo remission stage

Time of test administration	*Glycerol test	*Electrocochleogram	Furosemide tests: *Pendular rotation stimuli	Furosemide tests: Caloric stimuli
During vertigo attack	65% (31/48)	86% (18/21)	63% (5/8)	56% (5/9)
During remission stage	30% (14/47)	56% (15/27)	20% (4/20)	39% (9/23)

Numbers in parentheses represent the number of positive cases per total number of cases tested
$^*P < 0.05$ (X^2 – test)

Comparison with the Vertigo Remission Stage

A comparison of the rates for the two stages is shown in Table 16.4. The rates of positive results for the glycerol test were 65% during vertigo attacks and 30% during the vertigo remission stage. The rates of positive responses on the ECochG were 86% during the vertigo attacks stage and 56% during the vertigo remission stage. The rates for the furosemide test with centric & eccentric pendular rotation stimuli were 63% and 20%, respectively. Thus, the rates for all three tests during vertigo attacks were significantly higher. The rates of positive results for the furosemide test with caloric stimuli were 56% during vertigo attacks and 39% during the vertigo remission stage, with the vertigo attack stage showing a significantly higher positive rate.

Diagnosis of the Endolymphatic Hydrops Aspect of Ménière's Disease

Sixteen out of 26 patients (61%) with Ménière's disease reacted positively to the glycerol test. Sixteen out of 22 patients (73%) with Ménière's disease showed a positive response on the ECochG. The rate for patients with Ménière's disease who showed a positive response to both the glycerol test and the ECochG was high (82% or 18 out of 22 patients). Nine out of 26 patients (35%) with Ménière's disease reacted positively to the furosemide test with centric & eccentric pendular rotation stimuli. Finally, 13 out of 26 patients (50%) with Ménière's disease showed positive results for the furosemide test with caloric stimuli. In all four tests, the rates of positive test results for the cochlear system were higher than those for the vestibular system (Table 16.5). In the group of confirmed Ménière's disease, 11 out of 20 patients (55%) showed positive results for both the cochlear and the vestibular system. Five patients (25%) were positive for only the cochlear system, and three patients (15%) for only the vestibular system. In the group of suspected Ménière's disease, one out of six patients (17%) was positive for both the cochlear and the vestibular systems. Two patients (33%) were positive for only the cochlear system, while two patients were positive for only the vestibular system (Table 16.5). These results show that the rates of positive responses for both the cochlear and the

Table 16.5. Diagnosis of the endolymphatic hydrops aspect of Ménière's disease

Cases		Cochlear system		Vestibular system Furosemide test	
		Glycerol test	Electro-cochleogram	Pendular rotation stimuli	Caloric stimuli
Clinical diagnosis		Cochlea		Statoconial organ	Semicircular canal
1. Y.W.	MD	●	●	○	○
2. K.H.	MD	○	○	●	○
3. E.M.	MD	○	○	○	○
4. H.K.	MD	●	—	○	○
5. Y.T.	M′ D	○	●	○	○
6. H.Y.	M′ D	○	○	○	○
7. I.M.	M′ D	●	●	○	○
8. A.M.	MD	●	●	●	●
9. M.U.	MD	●	●	○	●
10. N.N.	MD	○	●	●	○
11. T.K.	M′ D	○	○	○	●
12. Y.O.	MD	●	○	●	○
13. H.M.	MD	●	●	○	○
14. Y.I.	MD	●	●	○	○
15. K.M.	MD	●	●	●	○
16. M.M.	MD	●	●	○	○
17. S.H.	MD	○	●	○	●
18. K.I.	M′ D	○	—	○	●
19. S.H.	M′ D	●	—	●	●
20. C.U.	MD	●	●	●	●
21. M.O.	MD	○	○	●	●
22. Y.W.	MD	●	●	○	●
23. S.T.	MD	○	—	○	●
24. K.M.	MD	●	●	○	●
25. Y.F.	MD	●	●	○	●
26. H.K.	MD	●	●	●	●

●, positive; ○, negative; MD, confirmed Ménière's disease; M′ D, suspected Ménière's disease

vestibular system were higher for the group of confirmed Ménière's disease than for the group of suspected Ménière's disease.

Discussion

Positive Rest Results for Ménière's Disease

Comparison with Sudden Deafness Without Vertigo

The reasons we used sudden deafness without vertigo for comparison were that it, too, is an inner ear disease, and that some cases of sudden deafness with vertigo might represent the first stage of Ménière's disease. As many investigators [6–8] have reported in connection with the glycerol test and the ECochG, it was difficult to make an absolute comparison of the rates of positive responses for the two tests because of the different criteria. Futaki and Kitahara [5] reported a positive rate of 88% for the furosemide test with caloric stimuli, higher than ours. This discrepancy could be explained by the fact that most of our patients underwent the furosemide test with caloric stimuli during the vertigo remission stage. In fact, for the patients who were subjected to the furosemide test with caloric stimuli during vertigo attacks, the positive rate was higher: 56%. We are not aware of any reports on the glycerol tests, the ECochGs and the furosemide tests with caloric stimuli and/or centric & eccentric pendular rotation stimuli performed on cases of sudden deafness without vertigo. Since the group with Ménière's disease showed significantly higher positive response rates for almost all the tests than did the group with sudden deafness without vertigo, it was assumed that sudden deafness, in spite of being an inner ear disease, is doubtfully related to endolymphatic hydrops, but that Ménière's disease have some direct relationship with this disorder.

Comparison with Suspected Ménière's Disease

It was to be expected that the group with confirmed Ménière's disease would have a higher positive response rate than the group with suspected Ménière's disease for the glycerol test, the electrochleogram (ECochG) and the furosemide tests with centric & eccentric pendular rotation stimuli. The reason why the group with suspected Ménière's disease had a higher positive response rate than the group with confirmed Ménière's disease for the furosemide test with caloric stimuli was presumed to be that more of the patients with suspected Ménière's disease had undergone the test during vertigo attacks. Since even the group with suspected Ménière's disease showed higher positive response rates for all the tests than did the group with sudden deafness without vertigo, it was concluded that there is a firm relationship between Ménière's disease and endolymphatic hydrops.

Comparison Between Vertigo Attacks and the Remission Stage

No reports appear to have been published comparing the positive response rates for the glycerol test and the ECochG performed on patients with Ménière's disease during vertigo attacks with test response rates obtained during the vertigo remission stage. In our study, the positive response rates for the glycerol test and ECochG performed during vertigo attacks were significantly higher than those obtained during the vertigo remission stage. The reason for this was assumed to be that endolymphatic hydrops generally progressed faster during vertigo attacks and that endolymphatic hydrops developed not only in the vestibular but also in the cochlear system. The positive response rate on the ECochGs taken during the remission stage was also high but the reason for this remains unclear.

Matsunaga et al. [9] reported positive response rates of 64% for the furosemide tests with centric and eccentric pendular rotation stimuli during vertigo attacks and 10% during the remission stage. Those results are similar to ours. The difference between the positive response rates for the furosemide tests with caloric stimuli performed during vertigo attacks and during the vertigo remission stage was smaller than those for the other tests. The reason was assumed to be that the caloric test was influenced not only by the function of the semicircular canal but also by that of the vestibular nerve, and that the test had a tendency to remain positive once the damage had occurred. Since the positive response rate for Ménière's disease, even in the vertigo remission stage, was higher than that for sudden deafness without vertigo, it was seen as further evidence of a relationship between Ménière's disease and endolympatic hydrops.

Diagnosis of the Endolymphatic Hydrops Aspect of Ménière's Disease

We hypothesized that positive response rates of the glycerol test and the ECochG revealed hydrops in the cochlea, that positive response rates of the furosemide test with pendular rotation test revealed hydrops in the statoconial organ, and that positive response rates of the furosemide test with caloric stimuli revealed hydrops in the semicircular canal. It was suspected that the positive response rates for the vestibular system were lower than those for the cochlear system because more of the patients underwent the furosemide tests during the vertigo remission stage. Aso et al. [7] reported that the rate for simultaneous positive responses to both the glycerol test and the ECochG was low (30%), perhaps because the positive findings for the glycerol test and the ECochG were slightly different. In our study, the rate was high (82%). Since the rate of the patients who showed positive findings for both the cochlear and the vestibular systems was higher than that for positive responses in either the cochlear system or the vestibular system, the results were in agreement with the clinical diagnoses. It could therefore be established that the diagnosis of the endolymphatic hydrops aspect of Ménière's disease supports the clinical diagnosis. Endolymphatic hydrops often occurred only in the cochlea or the vestibule. In the present study, we performed the four tests during almost the same period, but the positive response rates were extremely low because the tests were administered essentially during the vertigo remission stage.

Conclusion

We performed the four tests for Ménière's disease with patients with sudden deafness without vertigo as a control group and obtained the following results. The group with Ménière's disease had significantly higher positive response rates than the group with sudden deafness without vertigo for all the tests except for the furosemide test with caloric stimuli. The group with confirmed Ménière's disease had higher positive response rates than the group with suspected Ménière's disease for all the tests except for the furosemide test with caloric stimuli. The patients with Ménière's disease had significantly higher positive response rates during vertigo attacks than during the vertigo remission stage for all the tests except for the furosemide test with caloric stimuli. The diagnosis of the endolymphatic hydrops aspect of Ménière's disease proved to be useful for distinguishing confirmed Ménière's disease from suspected Ménière's disease.

References

1. Yamakawa K (1938) Über die pathologische Veränderung bei einem Ménière-Kranken. Otolaryngol Jpn 44:2310–2312
2. Hallpike CS, Cairns H (1938) Observations on the pathology of Ménière's syndrome. J Laryngol Otol 53:625–655
3. Klockhoff I, Lindblom U (1966) Endolymphatic hydrops revealed by glycerol test. Acta Otolaryngol (Stockh) 61:459–462
4. Okumura S, Matsunaga T, Matsunaga T, Naito T (1980) Furosemide test for Ménière's disease: Using centric and eccentric pendular rotation test (in Japanese). Pract Otol (Kyoto) 73:259–263
5. Futaki T, Kitahara M (1971) Furosemide (Lasix) test (in Japanese). Pract Otol (Kyoto) 64:373–389
6. Kobayashi Y, Yagi T, Aoki H, Ueno H, Inoue H, Kamio T (1986) Time course of positive reaction in glycerol test (in Japanese). Pract Otol (Kyoto) 79:711–715
7. Aso S, Mizukoshi K, Oi H, Ueda S, Shibuya T, Nagasaki T, Yoshida Y, Watanabe Y (1986) Transtympanic electrocochleography and the glycerol dehydration test in Ménière's disease (in Japanese). Pract Otol (Kyoto) 79:242–248
8. Mori N, Matsunaga T, Asai H, Suizu Y (1982) Electrocochleography in the diagnosis of endolymphatic hydrops (in Japanese). Pract Otol (Kyoto) 75:1254–1258
9. Matsunaga T, Okumura S, Suizu Y (1981) "Furosemide test" and glycerol test conducted in Ménière's disease patients: differences between attack and remission periods (in Japanese). J Nara Med Assoc 32:61–67

Chapter 17

The Significance of the Furosemide VOR Test for Ménière's Disease

Kanemasa Mizukoshi, Yukio Watanabe, Hideto Kobayashi, and Hideo Shojaku

Ménière's disease is characterized by episodic vertigo, tinnitus, and fluctuating hearing loss. It is generally accepted that these symptoms are closely related to the presence of endolymphatic hydrops in the inner ear [1, 2]. Hitherto, the glycerol test and/or electrocochleography (ECochG) have been widely applied for the detection of cochlear hydrops [3, 4]. Recently, a new caloric test using furosemide was developed for the detection of vestibular hydrops [5]. For the latter, however, there are occasional side effects such as nausea and vomiting which make the test difficult to use .

In order to detect vestibular hydrops without side effects, the authors have developed a new furosemide VOR (vestibulo-ocular reflex) test by using a sinusoidal rotation with computer analysis [6, 7]. In this paper, the new furosemide VOR test will be introduced. Its results will be analyzed in comparison to those of the glycerol test and the ECochG with regard to the detection of endolymphatic hydrops in Ménière's disease.

Materials and Methods

Materials

Eleven normal subjects and 89 patients with peripheral vestibular disorders participated in this study. Patients with peripheral vestibular disorders consisted of 43 cases of confirmed unilateral Ménière's disease, 21 cases of suspected unilateral Ménière's disease, 17 cases of delayed endolymphatic hydrops and 8 cases of labyrinthine syphilis. For diagnosing the above diseases, criteria adopted by Ménière's Disease (1975) and Vestibular Disorders Research Committee (1981) were applied [8, 9].

The Furosemide VOR Test

The VOR test was performed immediately before and 30, 60 and 90 minutes after intravenous administration of 20 mg of furosemide [7]. In this test, a subject with eyes closed was rotated sinusoidally for a period of 10 sec (0.1 Hz) with an amplitude of 120°. With a mini-computer (PDP11/34), the VOR was evaluated at each interval mentioned above by calculating the percentile of VOR directional preponderance (VOR-DP% [6]) i.e., asymmetry response to the rotation expressed by the following formula:

$$\text{VOR-DP\%} = \frac{\text{slow phase velocity (L)} - \text{slow phase velocity (R)}}{\text{slow phase velocity (L)} + \text{slow phase velocity (R)}} \times 100$$

Where *L* is nystagmus directed to the left side, and *R* is nystagmus directed to the right side. The maximum decrease or increase (shift) of VOR-DP% after the administration of furosemide was calculated and compared with the findings before administration.

Glycerol Test and Electrocochleography

In the glycerol test, immediately before and 30, 60, 90, and 120 min after intravenous administration of 500 ml of 10% glycerol, pure tone audiometry was performed by the same examiner. The criteria for a positive test result was a threshold improvement of 10 dB or more in two or more frequencies. In the ECochG, acoustic clicks of 100 dB SPL were used as stimuli. The output of the cochlea was picked up by an electrode placed on the promontorium. A negative summative potential with a ratio of its amplitude to the action potential of more than 0.37 was defined as the Dominant Negative SP [10].

Results

Normal Subjects

The maximum shift of furosemide VOR-DP% which occurred after the administration of furosemide in 11 normal subjects is shown in Table 17.1. Since the mean value + 2SD of maximum increase or decrease (maximum shift) of VOR-DP% did not exceed 10% in normal subjects, a maximum shift of more than 10% was defined as positive.

Cases with Peripheral Vestibular Disorders

Case 1.

A 47 year-old male, with confirmed Ménière's disease in the left ear. The results of the VOR test before and after intravenous injection of 20 mg of furosemide are plotted in Fig. 17.1. A VOR-DP% of 18.5% to the left was observed before the administration of 20 mg furosemide(a), but 30 minutes after the administration the VOR-DP% had decreased to 3%(b). Consequently, the decrease in the VOR-DP% is over 10% and considered as a positive furosemide effect. In this case, vertiginous attacks disappeared and the furosemide effect reverted to negative after intramastoid endolymphatic sac drainage surgery.

Table 17.1. Normal range of the furosemide VOR test ($n = 11$)

		Increased or decreased after i.v injection of	VOR-DP% furosemide 20 mg furosemide
After	Mean	SD	Mean + 2SD
20 min	3.66	2.79	9.24
60 min	3.70	2.30	8.30
90 min	4.00	2.66	9.92

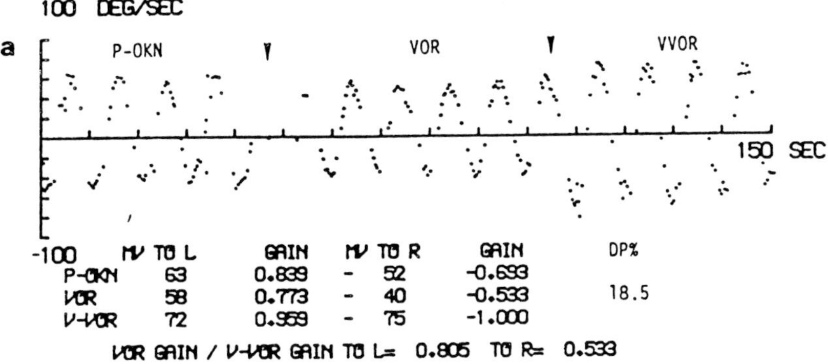

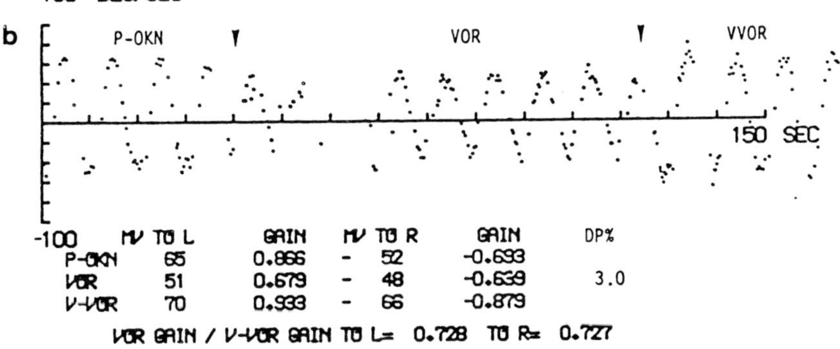

Fig. 17.1. Furosemide VOR test. VOR-DP% of 18.5% to the left was observed in a patient with Ménière's disease (case 1) before the administration of 20 mg furosemide (**a**), but 30 min after the administration the VOR-DP had decreased to 3.0% (**b**). *P-OKN*, pendural optokinetic nystagmus test with sinusoidal rotating OK stimuli; *VVOR*, visual VOR test with sinusoidal rotating in the illuminated OK drum; *Arrows*, light off and on; Ordinate represents the slow-phase velocity of the VOR, P-OKN and VVOR

Case 2.

A 20-year-old female, with delayed endolymphatic hydrops. She had been deaf in her left ear since around 5 years of age and had suffered repeated vertiginous attacks for several years. A glycerol test and an ECochG could not be measured because

Table 17.2. Incidence of positive results in the furosemide VOR test, the glycerol test and the ECochG in cases with confirmed and/or suspected cases of Ménière's disease

Examinations	confirmed cases (%)	suspected cases (%)
Furosemide VOR test(positive)	25/43 (58%)	12/21 (57%)
Glycerol test(positive)	23/39 (59%)	3/11 (27%)
Abnormal dominant-SP	27/40 (68%)	5/18 (28%)

Table 17.3. Response to 3 tests (furosemide VOR test, glycerol test and ECochG) in 37 patients with confirmed Ménière's disease in whom all 3 tests could be applied

		Vestibular Furosemide	Hydrops VOR
Cochlear Hydrops		+	−
Glycerol+	ECochG+	7	9
	ECochG−	5	2
Glycerol−	ECochG+	7	3
	ECochG−	2	2
Total		21	16

of the severity of hearing loss. The increase of the VOR-DP% after the administration of furosemide was 18%, and classified as positive. In this case, only by the furosemide VOR test could vestibular hydrops be detected.

Table 17.2 shows the incidence of positive results in the furosemide VOR test, the glycerol test and the ECochG in cases with confirmed and/or suspected cases of Ménière's disease. Table 17.3 shows the response to 3 tests (furosemide VOR test, glycerol test and the ECochG) in 37 patients with confirmed Ménière's disease on whom all 3 tests could be conducted.

Discussion

In the ECochG, dominant negative SP is often observed in cases with endolymphatic hydrops [11]. In the glycerol test, hearing improvement is presumed to be caused primarily by the temporary decrease of endolymphatic hydrops as well. In this test, however, caloric response results are not consistent. This may be due to the fact that this agent provokes direction-changing positional nystagmus in both normal subjects and in patients with Ménière's disease [12, 13].

In the furosemide VOR test, the shift of VOR gain may be chiefly caused by the temporary shift of vestibular hydrops due to powerful nutriuretics since no significant change in hearing is observed [5]. After the administration of furosemide, VOR-DP% decreased in some cases while it increased in others. The shifts of VOR-DP% after administration of furosemide could be divided into 2 types as observed in the glycerol VOR test [14]:

One is the shift of VOR-DP% decreasing the value of directional preponderance of nystagmus towards the healthy ear, and the other increases the value. The mechanism is not clear although it may be due to some biochemical alternation in the inner ear. The shift of both types are considered to be positive.

Compared with the furosemide caloric test, no side effects, such as nausea or vomiting, were observed in the furosemide VOR test. However, the value of the positive rate (58%) is slightly lower than that of the caloric VOR test (73%). In 2 cases of Ménière's disease who underwent endolymphatic sac surgery, it could be confirmed that positive furosemide VOR test results switched to negative after the surgery. In addition to the caloric VOR test, this test could be performed in cases where neither the glycerol test nor the ECochG could be carried out because of the severity of the hearing loss. In this study, findings judged to be positive for cochlear and/or vestibular hydrops were obtained in 94.6% of the 37 patients with Ménière's disease . This could be done by applying the furosemide VOR test can not be used as a substitute for them (Table 17.3).

From the above clinical observations, the authors conclude that the furosemide VOR test is as useful for detecting vestibular hydrops as the glycerol test and the ECochG are for cochlear hydrops.

References

1. Yamakawa K (1938) Über die pathologische Veränderung bei einem Ménière-Kranken. J Otolaryngol Jpn 44:2310–2312
2. Hallpike CS, Cairns H (1938) Observations on the pathology of Ménière's syndrome. J Laryngol Otol 53:625–655
3. Klockhoff I, Lindblom U (1966) Endolymphatic hydrops revealed by glycerol test. Preliminary report. Acta Otolaryngol (Stockh) 61:459–462
4. Yoshie N (1968) Auditory nerve action potential responses to clicks in man. Laryngoscope 78:198–215
5. Futaki T, Kitahara M, Morimoto M (1975) The furosemide test for Ménière's disease. Acta Otolaryngol (Stockh) 79:419–424
6. Ito M, Shojaku H, Kobayashi H, Watanabe Y, Mizukoshi K (1988) A clinical study of the furosemide VOR test for the endolymphatic hydrops diseases (in Japanese). Equilibrium Res [Suppl] 4:68–72
7. Kobayashi H, Ito M, Mizukoshi K, Watanabe Y, Ohashi N, Shojaku H (1989) The furosemide VOR test for Ménière's disease. A preliminary report. Acta Otolaryngol [Suppl] (Stockh) 468:81–85
8. Watanabe I (1976) Ménière's disease research committee of Japan. In: Morimoto M(ed) Proceedings of the 5th extraordinary meeting of the Barany Society in Kyoto, 1975. Jpn Soc Equilibrium Res [Suppl], Kyoto, pp. 281–283
9. Watanabe I, Ohkubo J, Ikeda M, Mizukoshi K, Watanabe Y (1983) Epidemiological survey of vestibular disorders (in Japanese). Pract Otol (Kyoto) 76:2426–2457
10. Aso S, Mizukoshi K, Oi H, Ueda S, Shibuya T, Nagasaki T, Yoshida Y, Watanabe Y (1986) Transtympanic electrocochleography and the glycerol dehydration test in Ménière's disease (in Japanese). Pract Otol [Suppl] (Kyoto) 8:242–246
11. Kitahara M, Takeda T, Yazawa Y, Matsubara H (1981) Electrocochleography in the diagnosis of Ménière's disease. In: Vosteen K-H, Schuknecht H, Pfaltz CR, Wersäll J, Kimura RS, Morgenstern C, Juhn SK (eds) Ménière's disease: Pathogenesis, diagnosis and treatment. Georg Thieme, New York, pp 163–169

12. Angelborg C, Klockhoff I, Stahle J (1971) The caloric response in Ménière's disease during spontaneous and glycerin-induced changes of the hearing loss. Acta Otolaryngol (Stockh) 71:462–468
13. Futaki T, Kitahara M, Morimoto M (1977) A comparison of the furosemide and glycerol tests for Ménière's disease. Acta Otolaryngol (Stockh) 83:272–278
14. Black FO, Møller M, Wall C III, Kitch R (1981) Vestibular and auditory responses to glycerol in Ménière's disease: Preliminary results. In: Vosteen K-H, Schuknecht H, Pfaltz CR, Wersäll J, Kimura RS, Morgenstern C, Juhn SK (eds) Ménière's disease: Pathogenesis, diagnosis and treatment. Georg Thieme, New York, pp 151–159

CHAPTER 18

Pathogenesis of the Broad Waveform in Electrocochleograms

Taizo Takeda, Haruo Saito, Izumi Sawada, and Masaaki Kitahara

The widened AP-SP complex is one of the characteristic features of electrocochleograms (ECochGs) in patients with Ménière's disease. This broad waveform has also been noted in other cases of endolymphatic hydrops, such as hydrops without vertigo, luetic hydrops, etc [1]. Hence, the broadening in the waveform of ECochGs seems to be of great value for the objective differential diagnosis of endolymphatic hydrops. However, a similar waveform is often observed in cases of retrocochlear lesions, such as cerebellopontine (CP) angle tumors and kernicterus [2, 3]. Since endolymphatic hydrops is not thought to be involved in these diseases, the diagnostic value of ECochG is thereby limited.

In the present study, ECochGs from 354 cases associated with vertigo and/or deafness were surveyed to re-examine the differential diagnostic value of electrocochleography. Additionally, two animal experiments were conducted to investigate the pathogenesis of the broad waveform in ECochGs in cases of endolymphatic hydrops and retrocochlear lesions.

Materials and Methods

Clinical Applications of Electrocochleography (ECochG)

A total of 354 patients with vertigo and/or deafness, including 164 with Ménière's disease, 19 with cochlear Ménière's disease, 8 with luetic labyrinthitis, 21 with sudden deafness, and 31 with vestibular Ménière's disease, underwent ECochG. ECochGs were recorded by a silver ball electrode placed on the posterior wall of the external meatus near the eardrum. Acoustic stimulation was presented at the rate of 8/s by a loud-speaker positioned 1 m in front of the patient's ear. The acoustic stimuli were 90 μs square clicks, and tone bursts at 2 kHz, 4 kHz and 8 kHz with alternating polarity. Responses to 1024 presentations of these stimuli were amplified and averaged with a signal processor (7T-11, NEC-SANNEI Co. Tokyo, Japan).

Animal Experiments

The effects of infusion of artificial endolymph into the scala tympani and the inactivation of cochlear efferents were evaluated to elucidate the factors responsible for the broadened waveform of the AP-SP complex of ECochGs. Normal healthy guinea pigs weighing around 300 gr. each were used for the experiments. All underwent a tracheotomy under general anesthesia by an intraperitoneal injection of sodium pentobarbiturate (25 mg/kg) and were artificially respirated. The bulla was opened ventro-laterally to expose the cochlea. ECochGs were recorded from a silver ball electrode placed on the surface of the bony wall at the scala vestibuli in the basal turn of the cochlea. The waveform of the AP-SP complex derived from this region resembles those seen in clinical ECochGs obtained by extratympanic recordings. Acoustic stimuli were 90 μs square clicks with alternating polarity, delivered at an intensity of 95 dB p.e. SPL through a loud-speaker placed 1 m from the pinna. Responses to 8 presentations of the stimuli were amplified and averaged with a signal processor (7S-11, NEC-SANNEI Co., Tokyo).

Experiment No. 1

In this experiment the waveform of ECochGs was examined when the artificial perilymph or endolymph was infused with 200 mm H_2O pressure into the scala tympani. Three guinea pigs were used for the infusion of the artificial perilymph, and three for the infusion of the artificial endolymph. A small hole (50 μm) was made in the bony wall of the scala tympani of the basal turn for the infusion. ECochGs were measured before and 10 min after the infusion, and changes of the waveform were compared.

Experiment No. 2

This experiment was conducted in order to examine the effect of inactivation of cochlear efferents on the waveform of ECochGs. Four animals were used in this experiment, including 2 control animals and 2 experimental animals in whom the efferent cochlear fibers were inactivated. All animals underwent a craniotomy to expose the cerebellum. After splitting the dura, the cerebellum was partially removed by suction to expose the vestibular nerve, taking care not to injure the cochlear nerve. In the experimental animals, inactivation of the efferent cochlear fibers was achieved by micropipette injection of 1% lidocaine into the root exit zone of the vestibular nerve. Control animals also received a sham operation to expose the vestibular nerve, but were not treated with lidocaine. The changes of the waveform of ECochGs were examined before and after the two procedures.

Results

Clinical Electrocochleography

The criteria employed to represent abnormality in an enlarged negative SP was defined as follows: abnormal type if the SP/AP amplitude ratio was over 0.37 in response to click stimuli at an intensity of 105 dB p.e. SPL; transitional if the SP/AP amplitude ratio was from 0.37–0.31; and normal if the SP/AP amplitude ratio was under 0.31, because 99% and 90% upper tolerance limits of the SP/AP

Table 18.1. Distribution of types of negative SP

Disease	Number of cases	Types of negative SP		
		Abnormal	Transitional	Normal
Ménière's disease	164	108	21	35
Cochlear Ménière's disease	19	10	2	7
Luetic labyrinthitis	8	4	1	3
Sudden deafness	21	8	1	12
Vestibular Ménière's disease	31	1	4	26
Dizziness	22	0	2	20
Sensorineural hearing loss	48	4	7	37
Tinnitus	9	0	1	8
CP angle tumor	6	4	0	2
Head and neck injury	5	2	0	3
Drug intoxication (streptomycin, kanamycin)	3	0	0	3
Otosclerosis	3	0	0	3
Otitis media with dizziness	3	0	0	3
Vestibular neuronitis	2	1	0	1
BPPV	2	0	0	2
TIA	2	0	0	2
Facial palsy	2	1	0	1
Parkinsonism	1	0	0	1
Harada's syndrome	1	0	0	1
Cerebello-spinal degeneration	1	1	0	0
Total	354	144	39	171

The diagnosis of Ménière's disease is limited to cases with recurrent attacks of idiopathic vertigo, sensorineural hearing loss and/or tinnitus. Cochlear Ménière's disease refers to cases of fluctuating hearing loss without vertigo. Vestibular Ménière's disease refers to cases with recurrent attacks of idiopathic vertigo without hearing loss BPPV, benign paroxysmal positional vertigo; TIA, transient cerebral ischemic attacks

amplitude ratio in normal subjects were 0.37 and 0.31, respectively. Table 18.1 shows the incidence of abnormal, transitional and normal types of AP-SP complexes in 354 patients with dizziness and/or deafness. The highest incidence of the abnormal type was found in Ménière's disease (66%). The incidence of the transitional type (13%) was not as low in Ménière's disease as in the other diseases. An abnormally enlarged negative SP, including abnormal and transitional types, was observed in 79% of patients with Ménière's disease. Cochlear Ménière's disease, luetic labyrinthitis, and sudden deafness also showed a high incidence of the same abnormality, 63%, 63% and 43%, respectively. This abnormality of negative SP was very rarely seen in the remaining diseases, except for CP angle tumor, which showed a high incidence (67%). The increase of negative SP in CP angle tumors was observed not only in response to click stimuli, but also to tone burst stimuli (Fig. 18.1).

Experiment No. 1

Figure 18.2 shows the comparison of the morphological changes of AP-SP complexes when artificial perilymph or endolymph were infused with 200 mm of water

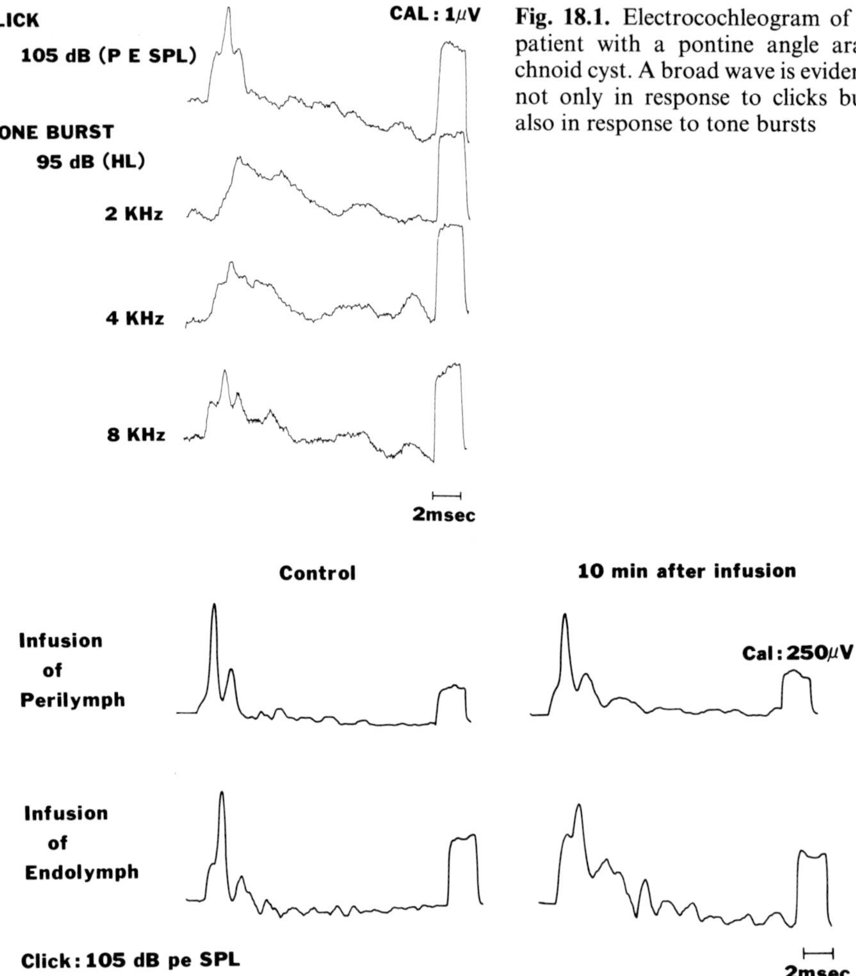

Fig. 18.1. Electrocochleogram of a patient with a pontine angle arachnoid cyst. A broad wave is evident not only in response to clicks but also in response to tone bursts

Fig. 18.2. Electrocochleograms with application of artificial perilymph or endolymph into the scala tympani with 200 mm H_2O pressure. Note the abnormally enlarged negative SP when artificial endolymph was applied

pressure into the scala tympani. The infusion of the artificial perilymph produced no remarkable alteration of the AP-SP complex. The infusion of artificial endolymph, on the other hand, induced the increase of negative SP 10 min after artificial endolymph was applied to the scala tympani.

Experiment No. 2

ECochGs were measured 10 min after the vestibular nerve was blocked by the injection of lidocaine, or following the sham operation. Figure 18.3 shows ECochGs from a control and an experimental guinea pig recorded 10 min after the operation.

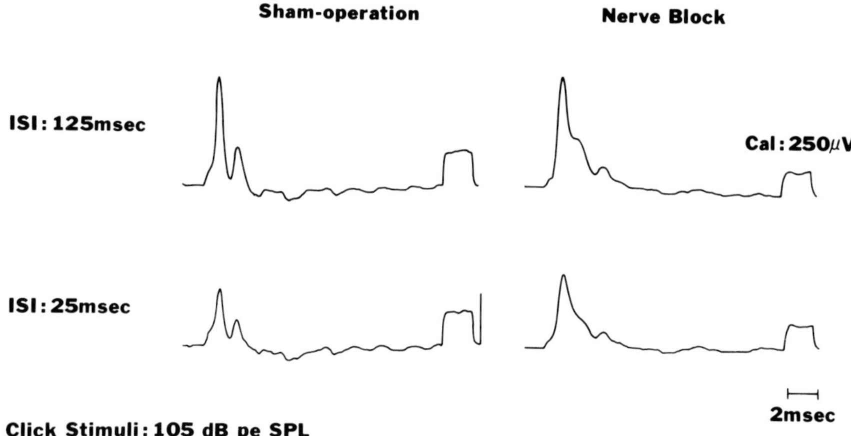

Fig. 18.3. Typical records of electrocochleograms in control and experimental animals. The sham operation induced no alteration of the AP-SP complex waveform, while inactivation of the vestibular nerve resulted in a broad waveform. Note that the broad waveform persisted despite the decrease in the interstimulus interval from 125 ms to 25 ms

The sham operation induced no morphological changes in the cochlear potentials, while marked widening of the AP-SP complex was seen in the experimental animal with inactivated efferent fibers. This broad wave persisted even when the interstimulus interval was decreased from 125 ms to 25 ms.

Discussion

The present survey of clinical ECochGs confirmed that the enlargement of negative SP is found frequently in patients with endolymphatic hydrops. However, CP angle tumors also showed a high incidence of the abnormal type of SP/AP amplitude ratio. This larger negative SP in cases of CP angle tumor, seen in response to tone burst stimuli, was morphologically similar to that in cases of endolymphatic hydrops. But, since CP angle tumors are not usually associated with endolymphatic hydrops, this abnormally enlarged negative SP is likely to have a different origin from that of diseases with endolymphatic hydrops.

The enlargement of negative SP in patients with endolymphatic hydrops has long been presumed to be derived from a shift of the basilar membrane toward the scala tympani [4], since endolymphatic hypertension is likely to be present, as suggested by the characteristic features of the temporal bone histology. Recent studies, however, have shown that there is no pressure difference between the perilymph and the endolymph, not only in normal ears but also in hydropic ears [5, 6]. Hence, the assumption of the basilar membrane shift is incorrect. Meanwhile, Dohlman proposed that the hearing loss in Ménière's disease was due to K^+ intoxication of the hair cells caused by leakage of the endolymph into the perilymph via Reissner's membrane [7]. According to this assumption, the perilymph contaminated with the endolymph comes via the helicotrema into the scala tympani, and consequently the increase in potassium in the perilymph occurs most significantly in the apical turn. Accordingly, the hair cells are presumed to be most extensively intoxicated in the apical turn, which results in a low-tone hearing loss, characteristic of that in early Ménière's disease. Furthermore, the K^+ intoxication also induced the increase of negative SP, as shown in the present experiment. The pathogenesis of the hearing loss in endolymphatic hydrops, including abnormally enlarged negative SP in clinical electrocochleography, could thereby be satisfactorily explained by perilymphatic K^+ toxicity.

On the other hand, a similar broad waveform of AP-SP complex was induced by the inactivation of the vestibular nerve, in which the cochlear efferent fibers run together. This broad waveform is also thought to be derived from an enlarged negative SP, because it persisted despite the decrease in the interstimulus interval. In general, CP angle tumors cause a variety of disorders of the cerebellum and/or brain stem; the efferent cochlear fibers in particular might be involved, as in the case of acoustic neurinomas. Therefore, it seems likely that the increase of the SP/AP amplitude ratio in patients with CP angle tumors may reflect an enlarged negative SP due to the absence of tonic efferent activity.

The SP, being a DC response to an AC stimulus as well as the product of harmonic distortion, is thought to result from the nonlinearity of the CM generators [8, 9], and this nonlinearity in the cochlea is thought to be closely related to the outer hair cell motility [10]. Application of solutions containing high K^+ is well known to produce a reversible longitudinal hair cell contraction [11]. Thus, the K^+ toxicity of the perilymph might influence the outer hair cell movement, leading to changes in the SP. Moreover, the cochlear efferent system may also control biomechanical nonlinearity by means of the outer hair cells [12]. Therefore, there is the possibility that the larger SP in cases of endolymphatic hydrops and CP angle tumors have the same origin with regard to hair cell function.

References

1. Kitahara M, Takeda T, Yazawa Y, Matsubara H (1981) Electrocochleography in the diagnosis of Ménière's disease. In: Vosteen K-H, Schuknecht H, Pfaltz CR, Wersäll J, Kimura RS, Morgenstern K, Juhn SK (eds) Ménière's disease: Pathogenesis, diagnosis and treatment. Georg Thieme, New York, pp 163–169
2. Portmann M, Aran JM (1972) Relations entre ⟨⟨Pattern⟩⟩ electrocochleographique et pathologie retro-labyrinthique. Acta Otolaryngol (Stockh) 73:190–196
3. Eggermont J, Don M, Brackman D (1980) Electrocochleography and auditory brainstem electric responses in patients with pontine angle tumors. Ann Otol Rhinol Laryngol [Suppl] 75:1–19
4. Eggermont J (1976) Electrocochleography. In: Keidel W, Neff W (eds) Clinical and special topics. Springer, Berlin Heidelberg New York, pp 626–705 (Handbook of sensory physiology, vol 5/3)
5. Takeuchi S, Takeda T, Saito H (1990) Pressure relationship between perilymph and endolymph in guinea pigs. Acta Otolaryngol (Stockh) 109:93–10
6. Takeuchi S, Takeda T, Saito H (1989) Pressure difference between endolymph and perilymph in a guinea pig model of endolymphatic hydrops (in Japanese). Equilibrium Res [Suppl] 5:88–91
7. Dohlmann GF (1980) Mechanism of Ménière's attack. ORL 42:10–19

8. Whitefield IC, Ross HF (1965) Cochlear-microphonic and summating potentials and outputs of individual haircell generations. J Acoust Soc Am 38:126–131
9. Engebretson AM, Eldredge DH (1968) Model for the nonlinear characteristics of cochlear potentials. J Acoust Soc Am 44:548–554
10. Kim DO (1986) Active and nonlinear cochlear biomechanics and the role of outer-hair-cell subsystem in the mammalian auditory system. Hear Res 22:105–114
11. Zenner HP, Zimmermann U, Scmitt U (1985) Reversible contraction of isolated mammalian cochlear hair cell. Hear Res 18:127–133
12. Siegel JH, Kim DO (1982) Efferent neural control of cochlear mechanics? Olivocochlear bundle stimulation affects cochlear biomechanical nonlinearity. Hear Res 6:171–182

CHAPTER 19

A Test for Predicting the Next Episode in Ménière's Disease

Jiro Hozawa, Fumiaki Fujiwara, and Toshio Kamimura

It would be very adventageous in the treatment of patients with Ménière's disease to be able to predict the onset of the next episode and possibly prevent it by careful management. However, despite extensive research, an exact marker to warn of an impending episode is still obscure [1, 2]. Alfero [3] reported the diagnostic significance of fullness in the ear, which could be evoked by the increase of endolymphatic pressure. However, according to Schmidt et al. [4], only half of Ménière's patients mentioned this feeling of fullness, and, in any event, this sensation did not always precede the attack. Other symptoms, such as increased occipital pain and changes in hearing are unreliable as signals for an oncoming attack of vertigo.

Uemura et al. [5] noted autonomic dysfunction durinng the Ménière's attack, and examined the pupillary response induced by the conjunctival instillation of Mecholyl. This investigation revealed that the pupil contraction rate was higher, particularly on the affected side, at the attack or quasi-attack stage. Pupillary change at the pre-attack stage was not reported.

We developed a computerized trapezoid rotation test to examine very minute pathological changes of vestibular function [6], and have monitored the clinical course of Ménière's disease by means of periodic repetition of this test. From the results of a six-year study, it was proved that this test had an excellent predictability rate for the onset of the next episode in patients with Ménière's disease. The method of this test is introduced and its result are discussed in this paper.

Test Method

All tests should be conducted in the dark with the subject's eyes open. Additionally, a number of question- and -answer tasks should be employed during the test to maintain the subject's level of arousal. All subjects sit on the rotary chair, which is accelerated by an exact trapezoid mode. [For this purpose, we used the Contraves-Goerz torque motor, DP300.] As shown in Fig. 19.1, after the 10 sec constant angular acceleration, the clockwise rotation is maintained at a constant angular velocity; then, deceleration is effected with the same mode as for acceleration. The magnitudes of acceleration and deceleration used in this test are 2, 4, 6, 8 and $10°/s^2$.

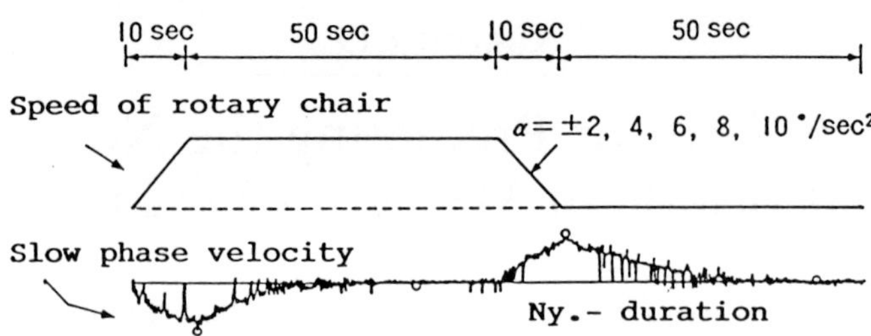

Fig. 19.1. Method of the trapezoid rotation test (see text)

The patient's eye movements during the test are recorded by electronystagmography (Fig. 19.1). The difference between the right- and left-beating nystagmus during rotation is calculated and plotted on the graph. [The automation of this procedure is made possible by a computer program.] The three graphs in Fig. 19.2 show the relation between the magnitude of acceleration and its nystagmus value. The abscissa of the graph shows the magnitudes of acceleration and deceleration, and the ordinate shows the difference of duration between the right- and left-beating

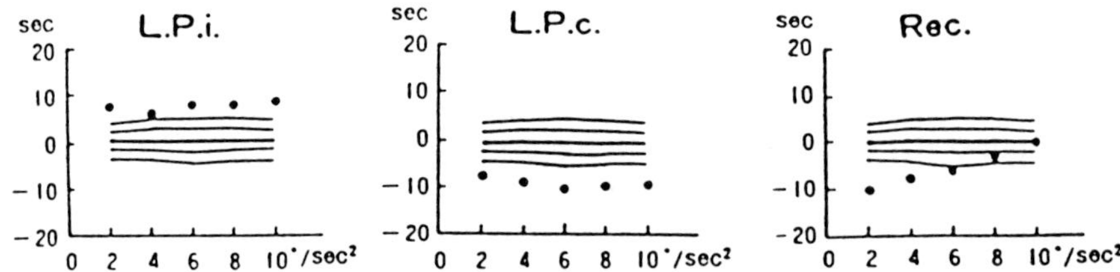

Fig. 19.2. Three abnormal types in the graph showing the relation between the magnitude of rotato stimulation and the test result (see text) *LPi*, ipsilateral labyrinthine preponderance type; *LPc*, contralateral labyrinthine preponderance type; *Rec*, vestibular recruitment type

nystagmus during trapezoid rotation. The five lines in this graph show the normal range obtained from 60 normal persons. The center line shows the mean value, and the other 4 lines show ±1 and 2 standard deviation, respectively. The data plotted automatically on the graph can be easily judged whether it is normal or abnormal.

Results

Classification of the Test Results

The test results obtained from Ménière's cases could be classified into a normal type and three abnormal types as shown in Fig. 19.2. The first abnormal type is the ipsilateral labyrinthine preponderance type ("LPi type"). This type originates from

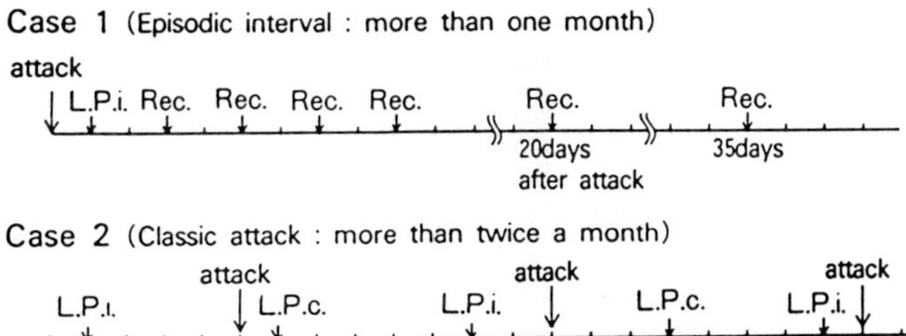

Fig. 19.3. Clinical course of Ménière's disease monitored by the trapezoid rotation test. One scale unit signifies one day. Abbreviations as in Fig. 19.2

the directional preponderance (DP) to the affected side, determined by audiometry and Fitzgerald-Hallpike's bithermal caloric test. The second abnormal type is the contralateral labyrinthine preponderance type ("LPc type"). This shows the DP to the healthy side. The third abnormal type is caused by the vestibular recruitment in the labyrinth of affected side ("Rec type") (Fig. 19.2). Finally, the normal type shows no significant difference between the right- and left-beating nystagmus.

Clinical Course of Ménière's Disease

The clinical course of Ménière's disease varies in each patient. As shown in Fig. 19.3, the stable cases without episodes for more than one month frequently showed the Rec or the normal type in the non-episodic stage. On the other hand, the unstable cases (with more than two attacks in a month) showed a type of labyrinthine preponderance. In these cases, the LPi type appeared frequently before the attack and the LPc type was common in the post-attack stage. (Fig. 19.3)

From these observations, it was speculated that the Rec type indicates a stable state of partial vestibular dysfunction on the impaired side. As long as this type is continuously detected, the attack is rare. But, when the LPi type comes to take the place of the Rec type, the attack appears frequently. Therefore, the appearance of the LPi type may be able to predict the next episode. On the other hand, the attack is frequently followed by the appearance of the LPc type.

Relation Between the Appearance of the LPi Type and the Onset of the Next Episode

In order to investigate the validity of the above-mentioned speculation, the following study was performed:

Twenty-three typical Ménière's cases diagnosed by case history and precise neuro-otological examination, were followed up by means of periodic repetition of the trapezoid rotation test. A total of 108 test results was investigated retrospectively to determine what "type" was detected before, during, and after the episodes. Figure 19.4 shows the relation between the timing of the testing and the type of test result. That is, until 11 days before the attack [B_4 in Fig. 19.4], the Rec type and

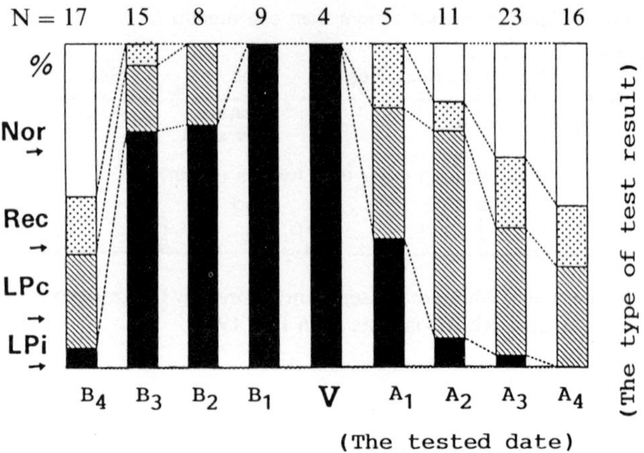

Fig. 19.4. Relation between the *date of testing* and the *test result*. The date of testing is counted retrospectively from the date of the Ménière's attack. The rate of each type tested at the same day is calculated as *percentage*. *Nor*, normal. Abbreviations as in Fig. 19.2

the normal type were frequently observed, while the LPi type was rare. Within 10 days before the attack [B_3] , the LPi type was prominent in the test results, and this tendency was more marked as the episode approached. Finally, no types other than the LPi type were observed on the day previous to and just before the episode on the day of onset [B_1, V]. On the following day [A_1], the LPc type was found in place of spontaneous nystagmus during the attack, and was the representative type during the several days after the attack. More than 5 days after the attack [A_3], the Rec type and the normal type began to reappear. From this observation, it was concluded that the detection of the LPi type was very useful in predicting the onset of the next episode. (Fig. 19.4)

Relation Between the Appearance of the LPi Type and the Development of Endolymphatic Hydrops

It is pertinent to explain why a Ménière's attack is preceded by the appearance of the LPi type. In some cases with Ménière's disease, we observed that the LPi type disappeared as hearing improved by the glycerol effect. Therefore, it seems that there is some relation between the emergence of the LPi type and the development of endolymphatic hydrops. In order to clarify this relation, 14 guinea pigs were examined by the trapezoid rotation test before and 2–4 weeks after obliterating their right endolymphatic ducts by Kimura's method [7]. Four weeks after the operation, a histological examination was performed on all animals. In this study, the LPi type was detected in 11 guinea pigs, in which endolymphatic hydrops was confirmed histologically. The other 3 guinea pigs did not show either the LPi type or endolymphatic hydrops. As shown in Fig. 19.5, it was concluded that there was a close relation between the degree of endolymphatic hydrops (classified by Paparella [8]) and the strength of LPi detected two weeks after the operation. Namely, more severe hydrops showed the stronger LPi (Fig. 19.5). However, as shown in Fig.

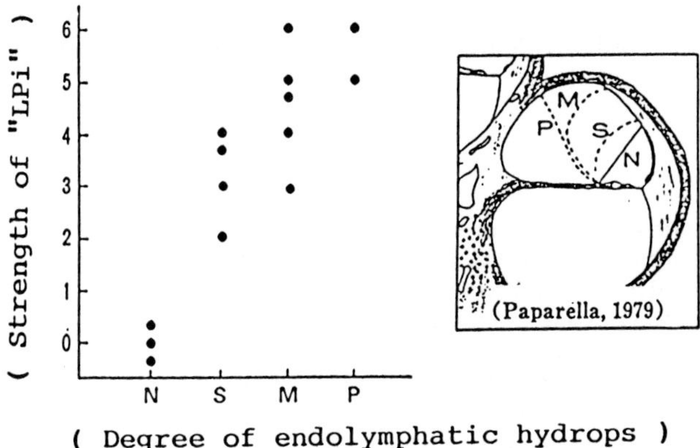

Fig. 19.5. Relation between the *strength of LPi* and the *degree of endolymphatic hydrops*. The ordinate shows the strength of *LPi*, which is calculated as the total difference of duration between the left- and right-beating nystagmus during this rotation test. The scale of measurement is the standard deviation (SD) of the normal mean value. The abscissa is the degree of *endolymphatic hydrops* which is classified by Paparella's method [8]

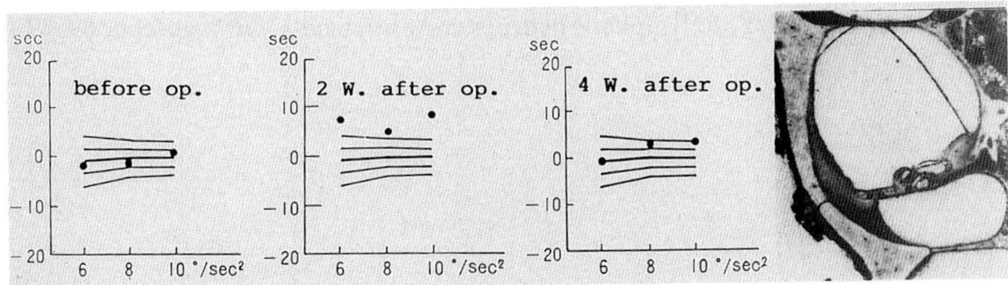

Fig. 19.6. Change of LPi after obliterating guinea pig right endolymphatic duct. Despite the severe hydrops (*right picture*), the strength of LPi detected 4 weeks (*W.*) after the operation decreased when compared with that measured after 2 weeks

19.6, despite the severe hydrops, the strength of LPi detccted 4 weeks after the operation decreased when compared with that found after 2 weeks ($P < 0.05$, Fig. 19.6). From this result, the appearance of LPi type was thought to be related with the speed of producing endolymphatic hydrops. It is possible to speculate that the rapid development of the endolymphatic hydrops took place immediately before the Ménière's attack. Therefore, it seems reasonable to conclude that the LPi type will be detected clinically before the Ménière's attack and is thereby a marker to predict the onset.

Conclusion

The ipsilateral labyrinthine preponderance (LPi) type, which was detected by the trapezoid rotation test, was proposed as a predictive sign of Ménière's attacks.

Seven of 10 cases, who were admitted in our University hospital and were treated by us in the stage of the LPi appearance, should be spared Ménière's attacks.

References

1. Watanabe I (1976) Ménière's disease research committee of Japan. In: Morimoto M (ed) Proceedings of the 5th extraordinary meeting of the Barany Society in Kyoto, 1975. Int J Equilibrium Res [Suppl] (Kyoto), pp 281–283
2. Mizukoshi K, Ino H, Ishikawa K, Watanabe Y, Yamazaki H, Kato I, Okubo J, Watanabe I (1979) Epidemiological survey of definite cases of Ménière's disease collected by the seventeen members of the Ménière's disease research committee of Japan in 1975–1976. Adv Otorhinolaryngol 25: 106–111
3. Alfero VR (1958) Diagnostic significance of fullness in the ear. JAMA 166: 329
4. Schmidt PH, Brunsting RC, Antvelink JB (1979) Ménière's disease: Etiology and natural history. Acta Otolaryngol (Stockh) 87: 410–412
5. Uemura T, Ito M, Kikuchi N (1980) Autonomic dysfunction on the affected side in Ménière's disease. Acta Otolaryngol (Stockh) 89: 109–117
6. Hozawa J, Fujiwara F, Saito H, Kamata S, Ikeno K (1987) The value of trapezoid rotation test by Contraves computerized rotary chair system. Acta Otolaryngol [Suppl] (Stockh) 435: 55–63
7. Kimura RS (1967) Experimental blockage of the endolymphatic duct and sac, and its effect on the inner ear of the guinea pig. Ann Otol Rhinol Laryngol 76: 604–687
8. Paparella MM (1979) Endolymphatic hydrops and otitis media. Laryngoscope 89: 43–58

CHAPTER 20

The Clinical Epidemiology of Ménière's Disease: Functional Asymmetry

Isamu Watanabe, Motohisa Ikeda, and Yasuo Niizeki

Acute or episodic vertigo is the most characteristic symptom of Ménière's disease. This kind of vertigo appears when the function of the vestibular labyrinth abruptly becomes asymmetrical. Therefore, a study of the origin of the asymmetry or laterality of a labyrinthine lesion is needed; it could provide one of the keys in solving some of the problems concerning the pathogenesis and treatment of Ménière's disease.

It is a popular concept that some kind of autonomic imbalance—especially in the head and neck region—could be an important factor in inducing a labyrinthine lesion. In spite of the wide acceptance of this idea, we are unaware of any report in the literature which has confirmed the existence of autonomic imbalance in the head and neck region with respect to the affected ear of Ménière's disease.

This is a report of our clinical epidemiological investigations concerned with the laterality of the lesion found in Ménière's disease.

Materials and Methods

In a series of clinical observations over the past 25 years, we found 12 cases of Ménière's disease occurring after surgery which involved the apex of the lung. Marked deformity of the area around the apex of the lung on the operated side was observed in all cases. The rate of these cases, among all cases of Ménière's disease, was less than 2%.

The diagnosis of Ménière's disease was made according to the criteria proposed by the Ménière's Disease Research Committee, Japan 1974 [1].

Results

Table 20.1 shows the list of cases of Ménière's disease occurring after surgery around the apex of the lung. The number of cases in both sexes was equal. The interval between the onset of Ménière's disease and thoracic surgery was 14.5 years on the average (range: 3–31 years). The majority of cases underwent surgery for tuberculosis of the lung. The type of operation was "upper lobe resection" (ULR) in 6 cases and "thoracoplasty" (TPL) in 5 cases.

Table 20.1. Ménière's disease and lesions of the apex of the lung: Age and side of lesion

No.	Name	Sex	Age at onset of Ménière's	Age at the time of op. or trauma	Interval (years)	Affected ear	Operated or injured side	Cause
1	S.M.	M	42	40	2	R	L (ULR)	TBC
2	K.M.	M	39	34	5	R	L (TP)	TBC
3	N.K.	M	40	35	5	R	L (TP)	TBC
4	O.S.	F	41	28	13	R	L (ULR)	TUMOR
5	O.H.	M	29	23	6	L	R (TRAUMA)	TRAUMA
6	Y.I.	M	55	24	31	L	R (TP)	TBC
7	S.S.	F	49	20	29	L	R (TP)	TBC
8	Y.Y.	F	40	30	10	L	R (ULR)	TBC
9	K.N.	F	48	34	14	L	R (ULR)	TBC
10	T.T.	M	64	34	30	L	R (TP)	TBC
11	F.S.	F	53	51	2	L	R (ULR)	TBC
12	M.I.	F	56	29	27	L + R	R (ULR)	TBC

ULR, upper lobe resection; TBC, tuberculosis; TP, thoracoplasty

Table 20.2. Ménière's disease and lesion of the apex of the lung: Laboratory data

No.	Name	Affected ear	Affected lung (use of SM)	Audiometry (dB)	Vest. exam.	Anisocoria	Diagnosis of Ménière's
1	S.M.	R	L(SM)	GH-40	SPN-L or R	$L < R$	Typical
2	K.M.	R	L(SM)	GH-45	SPN-R	$L \leqq R$	Atypical
3	N.K.	R	L	FL-60	CP-R	$L < R$	Typical
4	O.S.	R	L	LO-0	DEV-L	L ≒ R	Atypical
5	O.H.	L	R	FL-45	CP-L	$L \leqq R$	Typical
6	Y.I.	L	R(SM)	FL-60	CP-L	L ≒ R	Atypical
7	S.S.	L	R(SM)	LH-25	CP-L		typical
8	Y.Y.	L	R(SM)	GH-50	SPN-L		typical
9	K.N.	L	R(SM)	LH-25	CP-L		typical
10	T.T.	L	R(SM)	GH-30	CP $^{R}_{L}$		Atypical
11	F.S.	L	R(SM)	GH-35	CP-L		typical
12	M.I.	L(R)	R(SM)	LO-40(L) GH-25(R)	CP $^{R}_{L}$		Typical

GH, gradual high-tone loss; FL, flat; LO, low-tone loss; LH, low- and high-tone loss; SPN, spontaneous nystagmus; CP, canal paresis; DEV, deviation; SM, streptomycin; dB, average hearing level of the middle tone range

The most remarkable finding was the relationship between the side of the affected ear and the side of the lung operation; namely, the ear affected with Ménière's disease was always contralateral to the operated lung. There was one case of bilateral Ménière's disease but even in this case there was an asymmetry in the severity of ear problems and the most affected ear was on the side opposite the operation (Table 20.2).

Special clinical figures based on routine examinations such as audiometic or vestibular tests were not available. However, anisocoria associated with Horner's syndrome was observed in some cases (Table 20.2).

Discussion

It is well known that the majority of cases of Ménière's disease are unilateral. Additionally, even in bilateral cases there is marked asymmetry in the functioning of the two labyrinths. One of the leading concepts concerning the pathogenesis of Ménière's disease is an autonomic nervous system dysfunction. In spite of the wide acceptance of this theory, there have been only scant reports concerning the presence of autonomic asymmetries in the head and neck region of individuals with Ménière's disease.

Thus, a study was carried out to investigate the possibility of autonomic innervation asymmetries in individuals with Ménière's disease [2]. Of the patients with confirmed Ménière's disease, 129 were selected for the study in addition to 50 normal subjects as the control group. Asymmetries involving the following parameters were statistically significant when compared with the normal control group: blood pressure, skin temperature of the face, diameter of the pupils (anisocoria), and blood pressure of the central retinal artery. There was no correlation between the direction of those asymmetries (e.g., the side with higher or lower blood pressure, etc.) and the affected side in Ménière's disease patients. In some cases, however, fluctuations of these autonomic asymmetries corresponded to the course of the otologic symptoms and the episodic attacks of vertigo. In order to determine the possible cause of these autonomic asymmetries, the cervical vertebrae were examined roentogenographically in all cases. Distinct pathologic changes were found in the cervical vertebrae in approximately 20% of individuals with Ménière's disease, while in the matched control group, only 1.6% of cases had roentgenographically confirmed pathological changes of the cervical vertebrae. Other factors that may be responsible for autonomic changes in the head and neck region include middle ear inflammation, apical lesions of the pleura, and previous thoracic surgery, etc. [3].

Recently, it seems that local predisposing factors are becoming a matter of great concern for investigations as a possible cause in the etiology or pathophysiology of Ménière's disease. For example, there is roentgenographic (especially tomographic) evidence that underdevelopment of the endolymphatic duct and sac is present in individuals with Ménière's disease [4, 5]. Arslan [6] posed a new hypothesis based on the concept of a multifactorial etiology of Ménière's disease. He based this hypothesis on a large body of data concerning the varied and multiple histopathological effects that middle ear inflammatory disease can produce on the inner ear. The possibility that blast injuries induce certain cases of Ménière's disease was raised by Watanabe et al. [7].

In this paper, we have reported a new finding; the affected ears of Ménière's disease were contralateral to the diseased side of the apex of the lung. It is well known that postoperative, post-traumatic or postinflammatory adhesive changes around the apex of the lung produce asymmetry of sympathetic innervation such as anisocoria, differences in facial perspiration between the right and left side, etc. The majority of preganglionic sympathetic fibers exit the spinal cord at the T level, enter the stellate ganglion via the white rami communicantes, and then travel via the anterior loop of the ansa subclavia to the middle cervical ganglion. At this point, the close anatomical relationship of the ansa subclavia and the apical lung pleura is seen.

These findings recall the paper by Fowler [8] on the hypersensitivity of sympathectomized subjects at the time of application of epinephrine. In his experiment, not only the sympathectomized side, but the opposite side as well showed marked changes in reaction, and the various types of asymmetry appeared dependent upon the doses of epinephrine. It is not our intent to reject the excellent experimental study of Rambo et al. [9] which reported negative histological findings in the inner ear of monkeys after cervical sympathectomy. But we would like to suggest, according to the results of our clinical observations mentioned above, that it would have been advantageous to have given much more attention to the opposite inner ear and, in addition, to have had a much longer observation period.

Dr. Kidokoro, one of the senior thoracic surgeons at the clinic of the University Hospital (Tokyo Medical and Dental University) has collected clinical records of 1024 cases of lung operations performed between 1949–1973. He recently followed up 259 of these cases and, among them, found 7 cases of Ménière's syndrome (2.7% of the follow-up cases). According to the epidemiological survey conducted by the Ménière's Disease Research Committee Japan in 1977, the rate of Ménière's disease among the general population was estimated at 0.016%–0.04% [10]. By a simple comparison of these two percentages, the rate of Ménière's disease among patients who underwent lung operations seems remarkably high.

Finally, these clinical epidemiological findings recall the plurifactorical hypothesis of Arslan [6], who suggested that there are a number of interrelated etiologic and pathogenic factors which act simultaneously at both local and general levels. We agree with Arslan's opinion and hope to continue our study to explore new factors and their relationships with the origin of laterality of the affected ear in Ménière's disease.

Conclusion

Ménière's disease occurring after surgery involving the apex of the lung is one of the valuable models which illustrates a possible origin of laterality in Ménière's disease.

References

1. Watanabe I (1980) Ménière's disease. With special emphasis on epidemiology, diagnosis and prognosis. ORL J Otorhinolaryngol Relat Spec 42:20–45
2. Watanabe I (1959) Clinical investigation on the asymmetry of autonomic innervation in Ménière's syndrome. Jap J Otol Tokyo 62:2609–2635
3. Watanabe I, Nishida H (1971) Anisocoria in Ménière's disease. Equilibrium Res [Suppl] 2:71–78
4. Stahle J, Wilbrand H(1974) The vestibular aqueduct in patients with Ménière's disease. A tomographic and clinical investigation. Acta Otolaryngol (Stockh) 78:36–48
5. Kraus EM, Dubois PJ (1979) Tomography of vestibular aqueduct in patients with Ménière's disease. Arch Otolaryngol 105:91–98
6. Arslan M (1977) A new hypothesis on the plurifactorial etiology of Ménière's disease. Acta Otolaryngol [Suppl] (Stockh) 357:1–19
7. Watanabe I, Sainoo T, Tsuda Y, Shirotani T, Egami T, Dohi K (1968) Asymmetric blast injury of the ear and Ménière's syndrome (in Japanese). Otologica Fukuoka 14 (Suppl 1): 220–225
8. Fowler EP Jr (1953) Neurovascular hypersensitivity to symptoms and diseases. Acta Otolaryngol (Stockh) 43:271–280
9. Rambo JHT, Wolff D, Freeman G (1953) A research study of the effect of the autonomic nervous system on the internal ear. Ann Otol Rhinol Laryngol 62:1149–1173
10. Nakae N, Nitta H, Hattori Y, Maeda K, Komatsuzaki A, Mizukoshi K, Watanabe I (1980) Prevalence of Ménière's disease in Japan (in Japanese). Pract Otol [Suppl 2] (Kyoto) 73:1023–1029

CHAPTER 21

The Contribution of Otolaryngologists in the Diagnosis of Neuro-Otological Disease: Acoustic Neuromas

Masaaki Kitahara, Hiroya Kitano, Hirosi Tanaka, and Jouji Handa

An acoustic neuroma (AN) is one of the most important lesions to be constantly kept in mind when diagnosing neuro-otological pathology. In Ménière's disease, failure to reach a diagnosis at the incipient stage might be attributed to the lack of all the symptomatic requirements of diagnostic criteria. Acoustic neuroma, however, should be diagnosed at all stages. In order to evaluate the neuro-otological methology of otolaryngologists (ORL specialists), an investigation was made as to explore to what degree they contribute to the diagnosis of AN.

Methods

In 1989, a questionnaire was sent to all neurosurgical departments of university hospitals in Japan. Answers were obtained from 71 (89%) out of 80 departments. The form consisted of the following questions: 1) How many new cases of brain tumor did you treat during 1987 and 1988? 2) How many new cases of cerebellopontine angle tumor did you treat during 1987 and 1988? 3) how many new cases of ANs did you treat during 1987 and 1988? 4) How many new cases of cerebellopontine angle tumor and AN were referred from ORL specialists during the same periods?

Results

Table 21.1 shows the results of the investigation. The ratio of ANs to all brain tumors was 7.8%, and 48.8% of ANs were referred from ORL specialists. Departments in which a ratio of ANs to all brain tumors was more than the average of 7.8%, were classified as group A, and those of 7.8% or less were classified as group B. Departments in which a ratio of AN referrals from ORL specialists was more than the average of 48.8% were classified as group (a), and those of 48.8% or less were classified as group (b).

Discussion

According to the findings of the Vestibular Disorder Research Committee (1988), 46.5% of patients with Ménière's disease were treated by ORL specialists. Since a

Table 21.1. Acoustic neuroma (AN) treated at neurosurgical departments of 71 university hospitals during 1987 and 1988

Group	Aa	Ab	Ba	Bb	Total
University hospitals	21	12	16	22	71
Total brain tumors/2 years	106 (218–61)	105 (156–18)	105 (289–44)	105 (293–46)	105
Cerebellopontine angle tumors (avg. %)[a]	15.9 (28–9)	12.4 (18–9)	8.7 (15–1)	7.6 (19–3)	11.1
Acoustic neurinomas[a]	12.2 (24–8)	9.2 (12–7)	5.0 (7–1)	5.0 (7–0)	7.8
Cerebellopontine angle tumors[b]	54.2 (73–36)	19.7 (33–0)	47.3 (100–0)	16.9 (50–0)	38.6
ANs[c]	65.7 (83–50)	23.1 (44–0)	69.0 (100–50)	20.7 (42–0)	48.8

Numbers in parentheses are the maximum and minimum.
[a]Percent compared to total brain tumors.
[b]Percent referred from ORL specialists compared to total cerebellopontine angle tumors.
[c]Percent referred from ORL specialists compared to total ANs.

unilateral progressive sensorineural hearing loss is one of the first symptoms of AN and is often undetected by non-ORL specialists [1], more than 46.5% of the remaining patients with AN might have visited ORL specialists. In north America and Australia, before 1983, 68% of ANs had been diagnosed by other specialists. In above survey, the total exceeds 100% reflecting the numbers of both consultations and confirming opinions [2]. Therefore, AN which had been diagnosed by otologists would have been 48–64% of all cases. H. F. House (1989, personal communication) thinks that almost all ANs in the United States today are diagnosed by otologists, since most AN cases first present with hearing loss. J. Helms (1989, personal communication) feels that about 60% of ANs in West Germany are diagnosed by otologists since otological measures to confirm or rule out AN has tremendously increased during the last 15 years. In Japan, only 48.8% of AN cases were diagnosed by ORL specialists. It is very important for ORL specialists to be concerned with neuro-otological diseases, although it is not known whether or not this low ratio of 48.8% is unique to Japan.

In our survey, the average ratio of ANs to all brain tumors (7.8%) was almost the same as hitherto reported, and was considered to be reasonable. However, this ratio varied from 0% to 24% according to the department queried. The ratio could vary because 1) many patients with ANs might have been sent to departments other than neurosurgical departments in some hospitals, and 2) epidemiologically, the incidence of AN might vary in different localities. In the USA, of those physicians who limit themselves to otolology, almost all of them perform AN surgery together with neurosurgeons (W.F. House 1989, personal communication). In Europe, although a limited number of otologists perform AN surgery, each of them treats a large number of patients with ANs (U. Fisch, J. Helms 1989, personal communications).

In Japan, however, few ORL departments perform surgery on a relatively small number of AN cases. Since these hospitals were unforeseeably not included in this list, we presume that almost all patients with ANs were finally sent to neurosurgical departments in these hospitals (listed in Table 1). According to the reports of the Ménière's Disease Research Committee (1975) and the Vestibular Disorders Research Committee (1988), the incidence of Ménière's disease is greater in the western than in the eastern part of Japan. However, differences in the incidence of AN for various localities in Japan has not been reported. No geographic difference was found between groups A and B hospitals. Furthermore, the average number of all brain tumors treated in neurosurgical departments was almost the same (105–106 cases in 2 years) among groups Aa, Ab, Ba, and Bb. Therefore, the different ratios of AN to all brain tumors among hospitals cannot be explained by reasons 1) or 2).

Since the initial symptom of AN is unilateral progressive sensorineural hearing loss, we then tried to explain the different ratios of the ORL specialists' involvement in neuro-otological diseases. At hospitals in the Aa group, the average ratio of AN to all brain tumors was 12.2%, and 65.7% of ANs were discovered by ORL specialists. Clinical involvement of ORL specialists associated with these hospitals is considered to be excellent. At hospitals in the Ab group, although the average ratio of AN to all brain tumors was 9.2%, only 23.1% of ANs were found by ORL specialists. ORL specialists affiliated with these hospitals have found very few patients with ANs although many patients with ANs were found by other specialists associated with these hospitals. The involvement in diagnosis of neuro-otological pathology of these ORL specialists is very questionable.

At the hospitals in the Ba group, 69.0% of ANs were found by ORL specialists. However, the average ratio of ANs to all brain tumors was only 5.0%. Since the average ratio of ANs (7.8%) to all brain tumors in all hospitals investigated was reasonable, this low ratio in group Ba is probably due to the small number of patients with dizziness who visit these hospitals.

At the hospitals in group Bb, the average ratio of ANs to all brain tumors was only 5.0% and only 20.7% of ANs were found by ORL specialists. Clinical involvement of ORL specialists in this group seems to be deficient. However, the tendency towards a misdiagnosis of AN by ORL specialists in group Bb would be smaller than that in group Ab. Although much more information is required in order to clarify the cause of this variety of clinical involvement of ORL specialists among these hospitals, one interesting finding emerged: ORL departments in which senior physicians are active members of The Japan Society for Equilibrium Research accounted for 47% in group Aa, 37% in group Ba, 22% in group Bb and 0% in group Ab. There figures were in agreement with the ORL specialists' involvement discussed above. Interest in and knowledge of neuro-otological diseases seem to be decisive factors for causing the differences in the above ratios.

The average ratio of cerebellopontine angle tumors to all brain tumors was 11.1%. ORL specialists discovered 38.6% of these tumors, compared to 48.8% of the ANs. The degree of diagnostic involvement in hospitals by ORL specialists for cerebellopontine angle tumors was almost the same as those for ANs.

In this paper, it was revealed that the extent of contributions by ORL specialists to the diagnosis of ANs is rather limited and extremely varied among hospitals.

Not all ORL specialists are familiar with the diagnosis of AN. It seems to be easier for them to diagnose various kinds of neuro-otological diseases such as Ménière's, vestibular neuronitis, benign paroximal positional vertigo, etc., because the diagnosis is based primarily on information derived from medical histories. However the diagnosis of these diseases can be arrived at only when AN and other specific diseases are ruled out. The lack of knowledge and ability to diagnose AN means that there is also a lack of knowledge and ability to diagnose all neuro-otological diseases. This deficiency must be overcome by continuous and assiduous education and training.

References

1. Kitahara M, Mizukami C, Tanaka H (1989) Time of diagnosis of cerebellopontine angle tumor in relation to physician's speciality (in Japanese). Equilibrium Res 43:217–222
2. Wiegand DA, Fickel V(1989) Acoustic neuroma—The patient's subjective assessment of symptoms, diagnosis, therapy, and outcome in 541 patients. Laryngoscope 99:179–187

Part IV. Treatment of Ménière's Disease

CHAPTER 22

The Treatment of Ménière's Disease with Isosorbide

Hiroya Kitano and Masaaki Kitahara

It is widely accepted that endolymphatic hydrops is a common pathological feature of Ménière's disease. Therefore, at present, the most logical and effective medical treatment for this ailment is believed to be with drugs which reduce hydrops. Isosorbide (ISO) has been shown to be effective for glaucoma and intracranial hypertension, the pathologies of which are similar to that of Ménière's disease. In this paper, in order to determine the efficacy of ISO with regard to Ménière's disease, we attempted, in cooperation with 14 other institutes, a double-blind crossover trial of ISO on Meniere's disease.

Materials and Methods

The subjects consisted of 107 cases of Ménière's disease and 40 cases of suspected Ménière's disease, diagnosed according to the criteria proposed by The Vestibular Disorder (Ménière's Disease) Research Committee [1]. These patients were collected from the 15 medical institutes participating in the study. Of the 147 subjects, 70 were males and 77 were females, with an average age of 47 years. The study was designed as a double-blind crossover trial consisting of 2 contiguous periods of 2 weeks each (Fig. 22.1). The ISO was in liquid form and the Betahistine-Mesylate (BM) [2] in tablet form of the antivertiginous medicine, so the modified double blind mcthod of administration was employed (Fig. 22.2). Seventy patients were given ISO orally in daily doses of 90 ml (63 mg) divided into 3 per day, and 77 patients

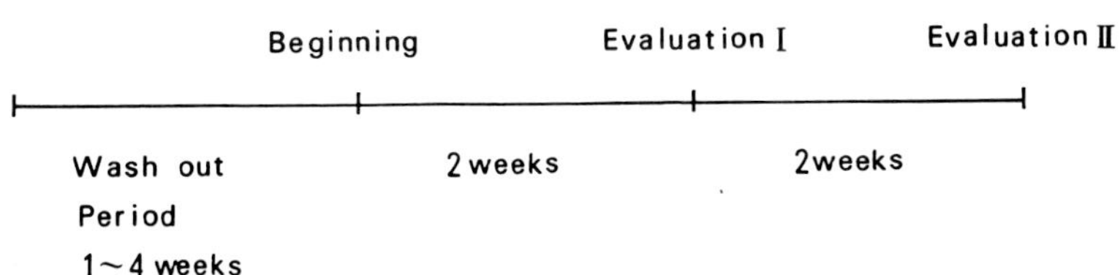

Fig. 22.1. Design of this study after a 1–4 week wash out period. The trial began. Evaluation was made at the end of the first 2-week segment and again after the second 2-week segment.

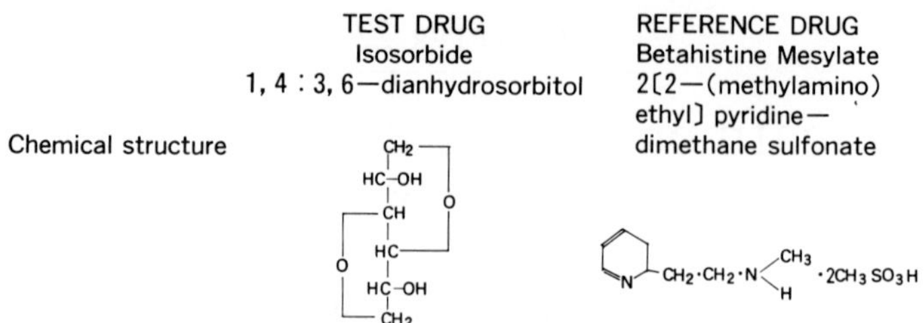

Fig. 22.2. Chemical structure of Isosorbide and Betahistine Mesylate

were given BM orally in doses of 3 tablets (36 mg) divided into over 3 times per day. The wash-out period was 1–4 weeks.

The effect of the medicines was examined at the end of the first 2-week segment of the trial, and again at the end of the second 2-week segment of the trial. Vestibular symptoms (vertigo and dizziness), cochlear symptoms (hearing loss, tinnitus, hyperacusis, and fullness in the ear), and erratic symptoms (headache, nausea, and neck stiffness) were evaluated on a 7-grade scale. Audiometric examination, equilibrium function tests and blood tests were performed at the beginning of the trial, at the end of 2 weeks, and at the end of 4 weeks, respectively. Glycerol tests were performed at the beginning of the trial.

A 5-grade scale was used in the evaluation of global improvement (an overall evaluation in change of prognosis induced by medicines) and the utility rating (computed on the basis of global improvement and the safety of drugs). The results of the examinations were judged independently by the attending physicians and the Judgment Committee (the Committee).

Results

Table 22.1 shows the results of global improvement of ISO and BM as independently determined by the attending physicians and the Committee. The attending physicians found a significant improvement greater in the ISO group than in the BM group both 2 weeks and 4 weeks after the start of the trial; the Committee, while recognizing the better results obtained with ISO, found no significant difference between the clinical effects of the two agents.

Table 22.2 shows the utility ratings of ISO and BM. In the attending physicians' judgment, ISO demonstrated significantly greater effectiveness than BM both 2 weeks and 4 weeks after the start of the trial. The Committee, while recognising the higher utility ratings obtained with ISO, found no significant difference between the two agents.

Table 22.3 shows the results of effectiveness of ISO and BM with regard to the various clinical symptoms of Ménière's disease determined by both the attending physicians and the Committee. ISO proved to be especially effective for dizziness and such erratic symptoms as headache, nausea, hyperacusis, and neck stiffness

Table 22.1. Results of global improvement with Isosorbide and Betahistine Mesylate

Judgment	Judgment period	Drug	Effectiveness	Significant difference
Attending Physicians	After two weeks	ISO	52/69 (75.4%)	*Positive*
		BM	47/76 (61.8%)	
	After four weeks	ISO	54/69 (78.3%)	*Positive*
		BM	50/76 (65.8%)	
Committee	After two weeks	ISO	49/69 (71.0%)	Negative
		BM	45/76 (59.2%)	
	After four weeks	ISO	52/69 (75.4%)	Negative
		BM	51/76 (67.1%)	

Positive indicates a significant difference in effectiveness, and negative indicates no significant difference. The ratios shown represent the number of patients showing global improvement over the number of total participants.
ISO, Isosorbide; BM, Betahistine Mesylate

Table 22.2. Results of utility rating with Isosorbide and Betahistine Mesylate

Judgment	Judgment period	Drug	Effectiveness	Significant difference
Attending Physicians	After two weeks	ISO	52/70 (74.3%)	*Positive*
		BM	49/77 (63.6%)	
	After four weeks	ISO	53/70 (75.7%)	*Positive*
		BM	49/77 (63.6%)	
Committee	After two weeks	ISO	48/70 (68.6%)	Negative
		BM	45/77 (58.4%)	
	After four weeks	ISO	51/70 (72.9%)	Negative
		BM	51/77 (66.2%)	

Positive indicates a significant difference in improvement rating, and negative indicates no significant difference. The ratios shown represent the number of patients showing improvement over the number of total participants.
ISO, Isosorbide; BM, Betahistine Mesylate

both 2 weeks and 4 weeks after the start of the trial. However, no significant difference was found between the effects of the 2 agents on the 3 principal Ménière's disease symptoms of vertigo, tinnitus, and hearing loss.

Positive glycerol tests and vestibular attacks occurring more than once a month were noted in many of the cases to be especially responsive to ISO, as judged by both the attending physicians and the Committee.

Discussion

The one consistent pathological characteristic of Ménière's disease is the presence of endolymphatic hydrops. This fact led to speculation that a hyperosmotic solution

Table 22.3. Results of effectiveness with Isosorbide and Betahistine Mesylate for various symptoms

Judgment	Judgment period	Vestibular symptoms		Cochlear symptoms			Erratic syndromes	Glycerol test	Spontaneous nystagmus
		vertigo	dizziness	hearing loss	tinnitus	ear fullness			
Attending physicians	After two weeks	N	P	N	N	N	N	N	P
	After four weeks	N	P	N	N	N	P	P	N
Committee	After two weeks	N	P	N	N	N	N	N	P
	After four weeks	N	P	N	N	N	P	P	N

P, significant difference in effectiveness with Isosorbide; N, no significant difference might be useful for both diagnosis and treatment of the disease. Accordingly, hydrochlorothiazide and a low-sodium diet with moderate intake of fluid has been used for treatment of Ménière's disease [3, 4]. Osmotic expanders such as glycerol, mannitol, and urea have been used in the diagnosis of Ménière's disease [5–7], but these agents have proved unsuitable as therapeutic agents due to such factors as the difficulty of oral ingestion and the pressure rebound phenomenon. ISO, originally employed in the treatment of glaucoma, was first used for treating Ménière's disease in 1980 by Kitahara et al. [8]; its effectiveness was subsequently confirmed by Larsen and Stahle [9, 10]. Although ISO was proved to be effective in reducing hydrops in animal models of Ménière's disease [8], large-scale clinical studies have not been reported. The present study is intended to fill the gap between animal experiments and clinical investigation.

Attending physicians judged that patients treated with ISO showed significantly greater global improvement than the BM-treated group both 2 weeks and 4 weeks after the start of the trial. The Committee, however, while recognising the better results obtained with ISO, found no significant difference between the two agents. The utility rating of ISO was considered by the attending physicians to be superior to that of BM both 2 weeks and 4 weeks after the start of the trial. In this case, too, the Committee recognized no significant difference. The difference in judgment between the attending physicians and the Committee members may be attributable to the fact that both the global improvement and the utility rating indicate an overall change in the condition of a disesae. The attending physicians were able to take into consideration the direct reactions of the patients, whereas the Committee based its judgments solely upon the data. Hence, while there were no major differences between the judgment of the attending physicians and that of the Committee with regard to individual symptoms, there were a few differences of opinion with regard to the general state of improvement in the patients.

In this study, ISO proved particularly effective for dizziness. In a clinical study, Kitahara et al. [8] found that ISO was effective for the symptoms of dizziness, headache, and tinnitus, findings which were later corroborated by Kitano and Kitahara [11] (both of these studies were open clinical studies; the present investigation was the first double-blind study to be performed with ISO). In the latter study, Kitano reported that a combined treatment with ISO and steroids was more effective than the use of ISO alone. In cases of tinnitus, for example, ISO achieved an effectiveness rate of 64%, but when used in combination with steroids, the rate rose to 84%. This finding suggests that in the treatment of Ménière's disease, combined ISO and steroid therapy might result in greater improvements in those symptoms which showed little response to ISO or BM in this study.

The effect of ISO on vertigo could not be accurately judged, since the short duration of the study precluded the precise observation of an intermittent symptom such as vertigo.

The attending physicians and the Committee were in agreement that patients with positive glycerol tests responded well to ISO. This is noteworthy, as ISO and glycerol are basically similar agents, although differences do exist between the effects of the two—the presence of the rebound phenomenon with glycerol but not will ISO is perhaps the best known example. Yazawa [12] suggested that these differences might be related to the drugs' molecular size in comparison to the size of the plasma membrane pores in the stria vascularis. The pore diameter of the plasma membrane is 8.0 Å, in comparison to the diameter of the glycerol molecule, 6.2 Å, and that of ISO, 7.9 × 3.7 Å. The small size of the glycerol molecule may enable it to pass more easily through the plasma membrane than those of ISO, providing a possible explanation for its quickness of effect. The size of the ISO molecule is much closer to that of the plasma membrane, slowing its passage through the membrane and possibly moderating its effect. This may account for its continuity of action and absence of the rebound phenomenon.

With regard to hearing loss there were no remarkable improvements in this study, a finding similar to that obtained earlier by Kitahara et al. [8] and Kitano and Kitahara [11]. Larsen, and Stahle [9], in contrast, reported that ISO therapy resulted in initial hearing improvements, a phenomenon also reported by another investigator [13]. Thus no firm consensus exists at present regarding the effect of ISO upon hearing loss.

In conclusion, ISO was found to be one of the few promising agents for the treatment of Meniere's disease, especially for its continuous symptoms.

Abstract

The clinical effects of Isosorbide, an orally administered osmotic agent, were investigated on 147 patients with Ménière's disease in a double-blind study. Betahistine Mesylate, an anti-vertiginous medicine, was used as the reference drug. The results of the study were evaluated independently by the attending physicians group and the Committee. The attending physicians judged the Isosorbide-treated group to be statistically superior to the Betahistine-Mesylate-treated group in both global improvement and utility rating on the basis of examinations 2 weeks and 4 weeks after the commencement of the trial. The Committee, while recognising the effectiveness of Isosorbide, found no statistically significant difference between the clinical effects of the two agents.

Acknowledgments. We would, in closing, like to express our gratitude to the other research facilities which participated in this study.

References

1. Watanabe I (1980) Ménière's disease. With special emphasis on epidemiology, diagnosis and prognosis. ORL J Otorhinolaryngol Relat Spec 42:20–45
2. Wilmot TJ (1972) The effect of betahistine hydrochloride in Ménière's disease. Acta Otolaryngol [Suppl] (Stockh) 305:18–21
3. Klockhoff I, Lindblom V (1967) Treatment of Ménière's disease. Acta Otolaryngol (Stockh) 63:347–349
4. Goodhill V, Harris I (1979) Peripheral vertigo and Ménière's disease. In: Goodhill V (ed) Ear diseases, deafness and dizziness. Harper and Row, New York, pp 526–544

5. Klockhoff I (1967) Glycerol test in Ménière's disease. Acta Otolaryngol [Suppl] (Stockh) 224:449–451
6. Klockhoff I (1975) The effect of glycerin on fluctuant hearing loss. Otolaryngol Clin North Am 8:345–355
7. Muskat J (1956) Urea in Ménière's disease and allied conditions; preliminary report. Arch Otorhinolaryngol 64:241–242
8. Kitahara M, Takeda T, Yazawa Y, Matsubara H, Kitano H (1982) Treatment of Ménière's disease with isosorbide. ORL J Otorhinolaryngol Relat Spec 44:232–238
9. Larsen H, Stahle J (1984) The effect of isosorbide and urea on hearing in patients with Ménière's disease. Acta Otolaryngol (Stockh) 412:113–114
10. Stahle J (1984) Medical treatment of fluctuant hearing loss in Ménière's disease. Am J Otol 5:529–533
11. Kitano H, Kitahara M (1983) Treatment of Ménière's disease with isosorbide and steroid (in Japanese). Pract Otol (Kyoto) 76:702–707
12. Yazawa Y (1981) Histopathological study of endolymphatic hydrops (in Japanese). Pract Otol (Kyoto) 74:2450–2506
13. Stahle J (1984) Medical treatment of fluctuant hearing loss. Acta Otolaryngol (Stockh) 53:258–263

CHAPTER 23

Transdermal Scopolamine in the Treatment of Vertiginous Episodes Associated with Ménière's Disease

Takeo Kumoi, Toru Inamori, and Hiroshi Mori

The parasympatholytic drugs, the antihistamines, and the phenothiazine tranquilizers all have a central depressant action and have long been used in preventing or treating motion sickness. The most widely used drugs are those with few atropine-like or sedative side-effects and thanks to the interest of the armed forces, many field studies and clinical trials evaluating drugs against motion sickness are available [1, 2]. In 1966, Brand and Perry [3] compiled exhaustive reviews on drugs used in motion sickness. They reported that there is no substitute for *l*-hyoscine (scopolamine) where the aim is to provide quick action but short-term protection against exposure to severe motion, but that for the prophylaxis of motion sickness during a long voyage, the diphenhydramine, cyclizine, may afford adequate protection.

However, although it has high efficacy, administration of scopolamine is frequently associated with side effects such as drowsiness, blurred vision and dry mouth, rendering this drug unsuitable for use on subjects who are performing tasks requiring alertness. To overcome some of the drawbacks associated with traditional scopolamine administration while preserving its efficacy, it can be given by a transdermal therapeutic system (TTS-scopolamine) recently developed [4], in which scopolamine is released for up to 3 days at a constant rate from a thin patch attached to the mastoid region. This has been marketed in western countries for treatment of motion sickness. Scopolamine taken orally at a dose of 0.3 mg has been proven useful in the prevention of motion sickness [5].

Vertiginous episodes of Ménière's disease associated with a unilateral vestibular lesion are different from motion sickness. Several drugs effective in the treatment of motion sickness have been tried in vertigo, because similar symptoms appeared in patients who were given cholinergic substances. The belladonna alkaloid blocks the synapse of the vestibular neuron at the nucleus [6, 7], as well as at the connections between the reticular formation and the vestibular nuclei.

Ménière's disease is a specific labyrinthine disorder characterized by episodes of true vertigo accompanied by transient hearing loss and tinnitus in the involved ear. The episodes of vertigo usually occur quite suddenly and are often very severe, frequently associated with feeling of nausea and vomiting. In some patients an attack may be preceded by an aura, which usually consists of tinnitus and/or aural fullness or stuffiness. We determined the beneficial and adverse effects of transdermally administered scopolamine on the vertigigo and nausea of Ménière's disease.

Patients and Methods

Twenty-one out-patients with confirmed Ménière's disease (10 females and 11 males with a mean age of 47.0 years) who could recognize relatively definite prodromal symptoms several hours before the occurrence of an intractable attack of vertigo, and who had symptoms of associated severe autonomic nervous system disorders were included in this study. They consisted of 12 patients in an acute phase (Table 23.1) and 9 patients in remission (Table 23.2). Written informed consent was obtained. TTS-scopolamine was applied retro-aurally when the patients in the acute phase group first noticed the aura of the impending dizzy spell, while in the remission group a sheet of scopolamine was applied every 5 days on the mastoid region. TTS-scopolamine is a 2.5 cm^2 flexible disk with an adhesive surface. When placed against the skin just behind the ear, the disk delivers a total of 0.5 mg of scopolamine (5 μg/h) into the systemic circulation over a period of three days.

The scopolamine release generally takes 2–4 h after application for an effective concentration of scopolamine to be maintained in the blood. Any concomitant use of drugs affecting the vestibular or vomiting centers, or the chemoreceptor trigger zones was contraindicated throughout the trial. In each case, otoneurological evaluations were conducted and subjective effects were reported by each patient who was asked to record all symptoms and adverse effects.

Results

Tables 23.1 and 23.2 list the two groups. The effectiveness of medication of TTS-scopolamine was graded as follows: marked or complete relief of vertiginous sensations, hearing loss, tinnitus, autonomic disorder symptoms and the objective findings of equilibrium test; moderately improved; slight relief; no change; and worse.

Tables 23.3 and 23.4 show the results and side-effects of TTS-scopolamine for both groups (cluster of attacks and remission). The feeling of vertigo elicited by Ménière's attacks was successfully alleviated with a patch of TTS-scopolamine in 10 of the 12 patients in the acute phase group, although the onset of attack itself could not be controlled. The same was true for the relief of the unpleasant symptoms of autonomic disorders in 10 of the 12 patients, but the cochlear symptom of tinnitus and hearing loss, and the objective findings of the vestibular system were only slightly affected by TTS-scopolamine.

Blurred vision and dry mouth were common complaints as side-effects. The tolerance was poor in only one patient who had a severe degree of dry mouth as well as blurred vision, while the other patients tolerated these side-effects. In the group of patients in remission, no significant effects on hearing loss or tinnitus were observed, and the side-effects similar to those seen in the acute phase group were present.

Table 23.1. Patients in the acute phase

Case	Age	Sex	Affected ear	History of Ménière's disease (year)	Interval between attacks of vertigo (Av.)	Unresposive to	Clinical course
1	56	F	Rt	14	4/1 y	Isosorbide Meclizine	cluster since the end of 1986
2	47	F	Rt	3	1/1–4 d	Isosorbide Meclizine	
3	43	M	Lt	3	2–3/mo	Isosorbide	cluster since Nov. 1986
4	41	M	Rt	3[a]	1/5 d	Isosorbide	temporary relief
5	39	F	Rt	5		Steroids Meclizine	cluster since March 1987
6	44	M	Rt	2	1/10–30 d	Isosorbide	
7	60	F	Rt	1	1/2 mo	Isosorbide Cobamamide	cluster since Jan. 1987
8	23	F	Rt	3	cluster since 1982	Isosorbide Diphenidol Betahistine	persisted dizziness since Feb. 1987
9	50	F	Rt	4	1/1 w	Isosorbide	cluster since 1986
10	38	M	Lt	2		Isosorbide	cluster
11	48	M	Rt	13	1/1–2 mo	Isosorbide	recurrence from endolymphatic surg.
12	51	F	Lt	5	persistent dizziness	Isosorbide	post sac surg.

[a]Disease history in months.

Table 23.2. Patients in the remission phase

Case	Age	Sex	Diseased ear	Duration of Ménière's disease (year)	Interval between attacks of vertigo (Av.)	Medication	Clinical course
1	71	M	Rt	6	1/3 mo	Nicardipine Ifenprodil	No attacks since 1985
2	45	M	Lt	3	1/2 w	Mecobalamin	No attacks since 1987
3	62	F	Rt	2	1/3 mo	Isosorbide	No attacks since 1987
4	52	M	Bil.	3	1/4 mo	Isosorbide	No attacks since 1985
5	37	F	Rt	2	1/1 w	Isosorbide Mecobalamin	Slight dizziness
6	59	F	Rt	20	1/3 mo	Meclizine	No attacks since 1987
7	30	M	Lt	1	1/6 mo	Isosorbide	No attacks since 1987
8	61	M	Lt	10	1/2 y	Isosorbide Mecobalamin	No attacks since 1987
9	31	M	Rt	3	1/3 y	Isosorbide Mecobalamin	No attacks since 1986

Bil, bilateral

Table 23.3. Outcome of TTS-scopolamine—acute phase group vs. remission group

	Acute phase group					Remission group	
	Vertiginous sensation	Hearing loss	Tinnitus	Autonomic disorder symptom	Objective findings	Hearing loss	Tinnitus
Marked or complete relief	10	1	0	10	1	0	0
Moderately improved	0	2	1	0	0	0	0
Slight relief	1	0	3	0	2	0	1
No change	1	9	8	2	9	9	8
Worse	0	0	0	0	0	0	0

TTS, transdermal therapeutic system

Table 23.4. Side-effects due to TTS-scopolamine—acute phase group vs. remission group

	Acute phase group			Remission group		
	Drowsiness	Dry mouth	Blurred vision	Drowsiness	Dry mouth	Blurred vision
Severe	0	3	3	0	0	0
Moderate	0	1	0	0	4	0
Slight	1	3	4	1	0	1
None	11	5	5	8	5	8

TTS, transdermal therapeutic system

Discussion

Scopolamine hydrobromide belongs to a family of natural alkaloids which was known to both the ancient Egyptians and Greeks. Preparations of belladonna have been used for centuries to relieve the unpleasant symptoms of motion and sea sickness. As extensively reviewed by Parrott in 1989 [8], scopolamine is the single most effective drug for the prophylaxis and treatment of motion sickness, although the effect of oral or injected scopolamine is rather short-lived, and leads to deleterious side-effects on autonomic and central nervous system cholinergic functions. TTS-scopolamine provides significant motion sickness protection, similar in extent to that provided by oral scopolamine or dimenhydrinate. The effects of transdermal scopolamine on motion sickness includng the laboratory investigations of simulation, are summarized well in Parrott's review and will not be reported here. Treatment of the vestibular symptoms with various anti-motion sickness drugs, e.g., scopolamine, dimenhydrinate, prophenazine, either alone or in combination with amphetamine or caffeine, has been recommended [9]. In recent years, TTS-scopolamine has been considered for the treatment of acute vertigo (Babin et al. 1984 [10], Rahko and Karma, 1985 [11], Lenore et al. 1986 [12], Pyykkö et al. 1988 [13]). Rahko and Karma [11] evaluated the effect of TTS-scopolamine and their double-blind study revealed favorable effects in Ménière's disease. In their study, the group of one active patch of TTS-scopolamine produced good or very good results in five out of six patients, and thc group of two active patches evidenced good or very good results in three out of six cases. However, Pyykkö et al. [13] documented a paper, in which, despite the fact that controlled, double-blind trials have already clearly indicated the benefits of scopolamine and dimenhydrinate on motion sickness, they did not have much data for the effects on vertigo in patients with Ménière's disease.

The present findings indicate that TTS-scopolamine is effective in reducing vertigo symptoms elicited by a Ménière's attack when applied just before or at the very beginning of an attack, although the small number of patients evaluated renders the results inconclusive.

As with other drugs for motion or seasickness, scopolamine, which is thought to act on both the vomiting center and the vestibular system [6, 7, 14, 15], seemed to be more effective when given prophylactically. In 1983 Kohl and Homick [15]

summarized the literature of neurophysiological data on motion sickness and reviewed the neurochemical and neurophysiological effects of scopolamine in relation to central cholinergic pathways, and concluded that the efferent nicotinic innervation at the primary sensory hair cells and the medial vestibular nucleus were identified as sites where modulation by cholinergic drugs might exert a beneficial influence. In fact, there are some reports on the effects of transdermally administered scopolamine on different types of rotation and caloric-induced nystagmus [2] and caloric-induced nystagmus [12]. Judging from the above mentioned reports, the controlling effects on the feeling of vertigo on patients in the acute phase presented here indicate that the site of action of TTS-scopolamine is on the vestibular system, and also that scopolamine has a strong anti-cholinergic action that can inhibit the vomiting center.

Finally, the application of TTS-scopolamine generally alleviates the adverse side-effects of scopolamine (blurred vision and dry mouth). When TTS-scopolamine is applied to the group to patients in the remission state, only the side-effects are influenced, without any change in the clinical symptoms of Ménière's disease. TTS-scopolamine intoxication in a 10-year-old girl was published in 1985 [16], followed by a report [17] of two cases (in a 12-year-old boy and 15-year-old girl) who experienced hallucinations with TTS-scopolamine. In using of TTS-scopolamine for Ménière's attack, it is essential to make the patient aware of the side-effects.

References

1. Graybiel A, Cramer DB, Wood CD (1982) Antimotion-sickness efficacy of scopolamine 12 and 72 hours after transdermal administration. Aviat Space Environ Med 53:770–772
2. Pyykkö I, Padoan S, Schalen L, Lyttkens L, Magnusson M, Henriksson NG (1985) The effects of TTS-scopolamine, dimenhydrinate, lidocaine, and tocainide on motion sickness, vertigo, and nystagmus. Aviat Space Environ Med 56:777–782
3. Brand JJ, Perry WLM (1966) Drugs used in motion sickness. Pharmacol Rev 18:895–924
4. Shaw JE, Bayne W, Schmitt LG (1976) Clinical pharmacology of scopolamine. Clin Pharmacol Ther 19:15–19
5. Wood CD, Graybiel A (1970) Evaluation of antimotion sickness drugs. A new effective remedy revealed. Aerospace Med 41:932–933
6. Shute CC, Lewis PR (1963) Cholinesterase-containing systems of the brain of the rat. Nature 199:1160–1164
7. Shute CC, Lewis PR (1965) Cholinesterase-containing pathways of the hindbrain. Afferent cerebellar and centrifugal cochlear fibers. Nature 205:242–246
8. Parrott AC (1989) Transdermal scopolamine. A review of its effects upon motion sickness, psychological performance, and physiological functioning. Aviat Space Environ Med 60:1–9
9. Balon RW (1983) The dizzy patient. Symptomatic treatment of vertigo. Postgrad Med 73:317–324
10. Babin RW, Balkany TJ, Fee WE (1984) Transdermal scopolamine in the treatment of acute vertigo. Ann Otol Rhinol Laryngol 93:25–27
11. Rahko T, Karma P (1985) Transdermal scopolamine for peripheral vertigo (a double-blind study). J Laryngol Otol 99:653–656

12. Lenore G, Schmitt RN, Shaw JE (1986) Alleviation of induced vertigo. Arch Otolaryngol Head Neck Surg 112:88–91
13. Pyykkö I, Magnusson M, Schalen K, Enbom H (1988) Pharmacological treatment of vertigo. Acta Otolaryngol [Suppl] (Stockh) 455:77–81
14. Jaju BP, Kirsten EB, Wang SC (1970) Effects of belladonna alkaloids on vestibular nucleus of the cat. Am J Physiol 219:1248–1255
15. Kohl RL, Homick JL (1983) Motion sickness, a modulatory role for the central cholinergic nervous system. Neurosci Biobehav Rev 7:73–85
16. Klein BL, Ashenburg CA, Reed MD (1985) Transdermal scopolamine intoxication in a child. Pediatr Emerg Care 1:208–209
17. Wilkinson JA (1987) Side effects of transdermal scopolamine. J Emerg Med 5:389–392

Chapter 24

The Status of Endolymphatic Sac Surgery

Masaaki Kitahara

Otologists who have no prior experience with Ménière's disease surgery must review the literature in order to decide upon the suitable technique for the case of the disease at hand. Until now, a wide variety of literature concerning modified techniques has appeared, suggesting that there seems to be no single technique which has satisfied any one surgeon. In most critical papers, the efficacy of conservative surgery, such as endolymphatic sac surgery on Ménière's disease, has been described as questionable because no significant difference from medical treatment has been observed. There was even an experiment indicating that the efficacy of an active operation to be the same as that of a placebo operation [1]. Is conservative surgery, then, really not effective for Ménière's disease? Additionally, is destructive surgery more preferable than nondestructive conservative surgery? In this paper, I will describe our policy of surgical treatment for Ménière's disease derived from 20 years of experience, primarily with intra-mastoid drainage surgery.

Endolymphatic Sac Surgery

Twenty years ago when I began surgical treatment for Ménière's disease, I reviewed the extensive literature [2]. Surgical technique for Ménière's disease could then be divided into 3 types: division of the VIIIth cranial nerve/labyrinthectomy, vestibular neurectomy/destruction of the vestibular portion of thc labyrinth, and labyrinthine decompression. Usually the former two types are called destructive and the latter is called conservative or nondestructive surgery.

Division of the VIIIth cranial nerve was indicated in cases with unserviceable hearing which could not be expect to improve. However, I did not feel that I wanted to jeopardize the possible effectiveness of any future treatment: I had been hopeful that the day will come when a revolutionary treatment for deafness will be developed. At the least, I didn't want to make it impossible even for a cochlear implant. Furthermore, since I already realized the prevalence in bilateral involvement of Ménière's disease [3], I thought that either ear could be a candidate as the only or better hearing ear. Ablation of the vestibular portion of the labyrinth seemed to be too sophisticated. Techniques for partial ablation of the labyrinth, such as electrocoagulation [4], ultrasonic irradiation [5], and cryosurgery [6], had been so rife

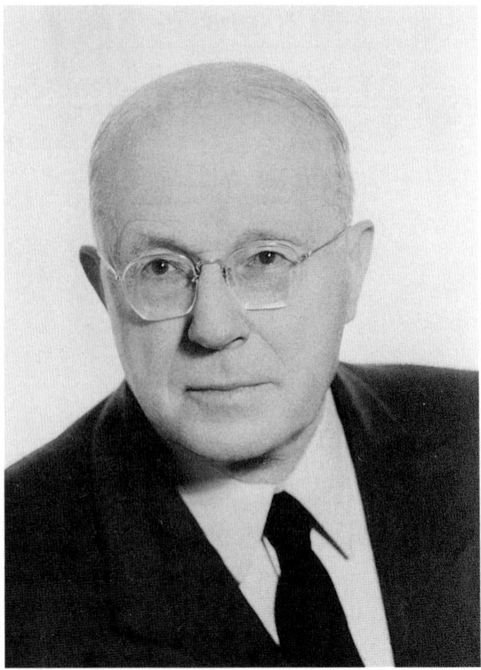

Fig. 24.1. George Portmann (1890–1985)

that one of surgeons performed the surgery for more than 90 cases per year especially using the latter two approaches [7]. Eventually, these techniques failed one by one and vanished during a short period of time. This alerted me to the fact that a valid evaluation of the results of this type of surgery, albeit so prevalent, requires a long period of time. At present, ototoxic drugs are administered by some researchers for the treatment of Ménière's disease. These drugs are expected to reduce endolympthatic production, but their primary effect is partial ablation of the labyrinthine same as with ultrasonic irradiation or cryosurgery. Any technique for the ablation of the vestibular portion of the labyrinth is always accompanied by the risk of the damage of the cochlea. Therefore, I am still reluctant to perform any measure directed towards even partial ablation of the labyrinth. When one wishes to remove vestibular function without eliminating hearing ability, I believe that vestibular neurectomy is better than any type of vestibular ablation at the labyrinth. However, the very low but not negligible incidence of total deafness following this procedure is a real concern. Furthermore, it is still doubtful whether or not the progress of this ailment could be alleviated by the partial division of the VIIIth cranial nerve.

Decompression surgery initiated by Portmann [8] was preferable to me for several reasons, especially the following: first, this type of surgery had continued uninterrupted for more than 40 years. Second, his initial surgery was believed to be harmless as he mentioned at the 78th Annual Session of the American Medical

Association in 1927. He stated "It is not dangerous and, therefore, can be attempted. If good results are not obtained, there is not any blame. If good results are obtained, very well". At that time, this statement had been confirmed by many otologists. Decompression surgery where the drainage was made at the cochlea [9–11], seemed to be effective for the control of vertigo but carried more risks for hearing than endolymphatic sac drainage. Ultimately, after some trial, we finally adopted endolymphatic sac surgery.

The major consideration for our selection of this surgical technique was the preservation of hearing ability.

Experimental Study on Intra-Mastoid Drainage Surgery

It had been noted that experimental studies on the surgical treatment of Ménière's disease, especially on intra-mostoid drainage surgery were conspicuously lacking. Then, parallel to the development of this technique, an experiment [12] was conducted on guinea pigs with the following results. 1) The endolymphatic pressure of guinea pigs with endolymphatic hydrops—developed by cauterization of the sac [13]—was not higher than that of normal guinea pigs. 2) When the endolymphatic sac was opened into the mastoid cavity after hydrops had been induced, Reissner's membrane was so folded back upon itself that the decrease of the hydrops was confirmed. However, the pressure of the cochlear duct did not decrease to 0 mm of water pressure, i.e., atmospheric pressure. The sensory epitherium in the organ of Corti appeared to be normal. Also, no abnormality was detected in the ECochG of the normal guinea pigs with open endolymphatic sacs. 3) The passage through the vestibular aqueduct was in one way only—from cochlear duct to endolymphatic sac—when the pressure was under 300 mm H_2O. When artificial endolymph was injected into the scala media through the wall of the stria vascularis with a speed of 0.02 μl/s, the endolymphatic pressure increased more slowly in the guinea pigs with opened endolymphatic sacs than in normal ones. This effect could be obtained only when the endolymphatic sac opening included the rugous portion of the sac. When artificial endolymph was injected with a speed of 0.08 μl/s, this effect was not observed.

These findings indicate that the vestibular aqueduct has some kind of regulating mechanism and that intra-mastoid drainage surgery would exclude any possibility of damage to the cochlear duct. The technique of the management of the sac will obviously influence the effects, and opening the rugous portion is necessary in order to obtain gratifying results. Since this type of surgery may have limited effect on the control of vertigo, combining it with other treatments, such as medication, is considered to be essential.

Development of the Technique

In 1951, Yamakawa and Naito [14] developed subarachnoid drainage surgery, and in 1961, House [15] introduced the subarachnoid shunt operation. These techniques were aimed at making a permanent hole in the endolymphatic sac. However, it was doubtful whether or not the drainage into the subarachnoid space provided an adequate suction effect on the endolymphatic fluid. According to our experiment [12], endolymphatic pressure in guinea pigs with endolymphatic hydrops was not higher than that of normals. If perilymphatic pressure exceeds endolymphatic pressure, as reported by Weille and O' Brien [16], this procedure may have the opposite effect on the elimination of endolymphatic pressure. Actually, when an incision was made at the lateral wall of the sac, we could not observe an immediate ooze of endolymphatic fluid in approximately 30% of all cases [13]. This finding indicated that endolymph does not pass freely through the vestibular aqueduct to the sac. If such is the case, a greater suction effect for adequate drainage has to be considered. Because of the above reasons, I preferred intra-mastoid drainage surgery instead of drainage to the subarachnoid space where the pressure is higher than the atmospheric pressure in the mastoid cavity.

After a while, however, I realized that Portmann's original method was not that effective. Therefore, I tried to expose the endolymphatic sac, including the rugous portion, as extensively as possible. The rugous portion could be identified by touching the posterior bony wall through it. The operculum was removed if possible. Then, a big hole which would not readily close was made in the lateral wall of the sac using a specific technique [17–19]. At present, I believe that making a new sac as large as possible alongside the pneumatic cells—which have developed in the post-operative mastoid cavity—must be the key to success, although it may be impossible to make a permanent hole in the wall of endolymphatic sac. These pneumatic cells are separated only by epithelium. For this purpose, a wide mastoidectomy is required in addition to appropriate management of the endolymphatic sac. There are many modifications of intra-mastoid drainage surgery. All techniques are supposedly intended to rebuild a sac with a large volume.

At an early stage of our Ménière's disease surgery, it was confirmed that our technique was more effective than Portmann's original surgery, Shambaugh's decompression surgery [17] and medical treatment [17, 19].

Present Status of Endolymphatic Sac Surgery

Although it has been confirmed through our extensive investigations that the efficacy of the newly designed intra-mastoid drainage surgery is superior to Portmann's original method and to medical treatment, many reports have appeared in the literature contradicting the superiority of this surgery. Some of the contradiction seems to be due in part to the fact that critics simply compare the results appearing in medical papers without noticing the differences in the characteristics of the patients composing each group, or they disregard the differences in minor criteria for reporting treatment results [20]. Usually, patients who undergo surgery have a longer-standing disease, more frequent attacks, and higher thresholds of hearing than patients who receive medical treatment [19]. Additionally, a larger percentage of patients who undergo surgery are older than those who receive medical treatment [19]. Over a long period of time, the hearing of the older patients would naturally become worse than that of the younger patients. It is possible that the above characteristics in each group more or less influence the level of efficacy of each group. Even when the criteria for reporting treatment results seems to be the same, the results are markedly different according to whether or not the definitive attacks which occur for short periods of time immediately following surgery are included in the calculation. Usually, episodes of dizziness occurring for short periods of time immediately following the administration of ototoxic drugs are not included in the calculation. It is important to re-examine the guidelines for reporting treatment results.

Even though surgical results are not very different from the results of other types of treatment, it must be recognized that a surgeon's impression obtained from his experiences will have a strong influence upon his attitude towards the selection of the technique of choice. Although they try to include every aspect of their surgical results in their reports, many aspects that they have perceived are unintentionally left out. As surgeons who have experiences with endolymphatic sac surgery realize, it is sometimes difficult to decide whether the moderated attacks following surgery are definitive or not. Differences in sensations of either spinning around and around for several hours and of feeling a slight streaming past of objects for several minutes have not appeared in any report. Are they recognized as definitive if the attacks are so severe that the patient is disappointed though does not deny improvement in his postoperative condition? Presurgical explanations by the surgeon are decisive as to whether or not the patient is satisfied with the moderation of preoperative severe dizziness or disappointed by the presence of moderated post operative dizziness. Patients who had strongly complained of head and neck dullness sometimes report that the feeling of ear fullness and the head and neck dullness are gone after surgery—as if they had received new heads and necks. These are not reported as results of either medical treatment or of other types of surgical treatment. On the other hand, even if morbidity of a certain type of surgery is low, the impact on the surgeon— from the complications following the surgery—can make him feel that it far exceeds the reported low morbidity. It is interesting to note that most surgeons experienced in vestibular neurectomy think that it should be performed when endolymphatic sac surgery has failed or only as a last resort. On the other hand, researchers who have no experience with this surgery often contend that the vestibular neurectomy is the technique of choice.

Thomsen et al. [1] performed a double-blind study concerning Plester's intra-mastoid drainage surgery. In their recent paper, they wrote that they believe they could handle the vast majority of patients with Ménière's disease by using a combination of symptomatic medical therapy, physical therapy, vestibular rehabilitation, psychotherapy, patience in listening to the complaints of the patient, and by convincing the patient that he does not have a serious, life-threatening disease. They selected 30 cases for surgery because the treatments listed above were unsuccessful as most experienced physicians have indicated. Thus, they obtained significantly improved results compared with preoperative scoring both in the Plester's intra-mastoid drainage and in the mastoidectomy groups. Nevertheless, they insist that they prefer vestibular neurectomy as their first choice of techniques. It is difficult for us to understand how they arrived at the above conclusions.

Comment on the interpretation of their results will not be included in this paper because a number of questions and criticisms have been presented by many other researchers.

It is very important to understand the limitations of intra-mastoid drainage surgery. If the vestibular aqueduct is narrow and obstructed, this type of surgery accomplishes nothing. If the endolymphatic sac including the rugous portion is not exposed, this type of surgery is less effective than other approaches, and because of this, the surgeons' skill is of utmost importance. It is generally accepted that the endolymphatic sacs of patients with Ménière's disease are small. Determining whether the sacs are small or not also depends upon the surgeons' skill. Experts can obtain good results; however if a new endolymphatic sac is required in order to deal with the excessive endolymphatic fluid, the surgery will be regarded as less effective according to the experiment mentioned above [12]. Therefore, it is preferable in selective cases which have good pre-conditions for the procedure, such as a visible vestibular aqueduct, a positive glycerol test etc., that surgery be performed by an expert. Additional medical treatment as well as psychological support are essential [19]. If episodes reoccur after considerable periods of time following surgery, revision is strongly advised. We have to reflect on the present situation where surgery is often performed by unpracticed hands (because of the low risk) on any cases which have only failed drug therapy and where revisions are not generally carried out even when indicated. It is, of course, absurd to restrict surgeons to only endolymphatic sac surgery. However, only otologists who are seriously concerned with the patient's hearing should be permitted to treat Ménière's disease.

After twenty years of experience, again we must conclude that an improved intra-mastoid drainage surgery is preferable—at least for the first choice—because it is an excellent physiological treatment with minimum complications and considerable benefit for a relatively larger number of patients.

References

1. Thomsen J. Bretlau P (1986) General conclusion. In: Pfaltz CR (ed) Controversial aspects of Ménière's disease. Georg Thieme, Stuttgart, pp. 120–136
2. Kitahara M (1971) Surgical treatment of Ménière's disease (in Japanese). Pract Otol (Kyoto) 64:349–369
3. Kitahara M, Matsubara H, Takeda T, Yazawa Y (1979) Bilateral Ménière's disease. Adv Otorhinolaryngol 25:117–121
4. Day KM (1943) Labyrinthine surgery for Ménière's disease. Laryngoscope 53:617–630
5. Arslan M (1953) Treatment of Ménière's syndrome by direct application of ultrasound waves to the vestibular system. In: Proceedings of the international congress of otolaryngology, Amsterdam, pp. 429–436
6. Wolfson RJ (1966) Cryosurgery of the labyrinth. Laryngoscope 76:733–753
7. Kitahara M, Kitajima K, Yazawa Y, Uchida K (1987) Endolymphatic sac surgery for Ménière's disease: Eighteen-year experience with the Kitahara sac operation. Am J Otol 4:283–286
8. Portmann G (1927) Vertigo: Surgical treatment by opening the saccus endolymphaticus. Arch Otolaryngol 6:309–319
9. Fick IA (1965) Sacculotomy for hydrops. Laryngoscope 75:1531–1546

10. Cody DTR (1967) Automatic repetitive decompression of the saccule in endolymphatic hydrops. Laryngoscope 77:1480–1501
11. Pulec JL (1968) The otoperotic shunt. In: Pulec JL (ed) Ménière's disease. Saunders, Phil adelphia, pp 643–648
12. Kitahara M, Takeda T, Yazawa Y, Matsubara H, Kitano H (1982) Experimental study on Ménière's disease. Otolaryngol Head Neck Surg 90:470–481
13. Kitahara M, Takeda T, Yazawa Y, Matsubara H (1980) Surgical confirmation of endolymphatic hydrops by hearing gain by bone conduction. In: Proceedings of the 6th Shambaugh international workshop on microsurgery and the 3rd Shea fluctuating hearing loss symposium. Strode, Huntsville, pp 260–263
14. Yamakawa K, Naito T (1954) The modification of Portmann's operation for Ménière's disease (in Japanese). Med J Osaka University 5:167–175
15. House WF (1962) Subarachnoid shunt for drainage of endolymphatic hydrops. Laryngoscope 72:713–729
16. Weille FL, O'Brien HF (1958) Pressures of the labyrinthine fluids. Ann Otol Rhinol Laryngol 67:858
17. Kitahara M, Futaki T, Morimoto M (1974) Epidural drainage operation for Ménière's disease (in Japanese). Equilibrium Res 4:48–51
18. Kitahara M, Takeda T, Yazawa Y, Matsubara H (1983) Experimental and clinical studies on epidural drainage surgery. Adv Otorhinolaryngol 30:242–244
19. Kitahara M, Kitano H (1985) Surgical treatment of Ménière's disease. Am J Otol 6: 108–109
20. Kithahara M, Kitajima K (1988) Intramastoid drainage surgery for Ménière's disease—Critical analysis of variation of surgical results for Ménière's disease. Adv Otorhinolaryngol 42:269–274

Part V. Other Diseases with Endolymphatic Hydrops

CHAPTER 25

Endolymphatic Hydrops Induced by Chronic Otitis Media

Etsuo Yamamoto and Chikashi Mizukami

Some patients with otitis media complain of symptoms characteristic of Ménière's disease (vertigo, tinnitus, and fluctuating hearing loss). Paparella et al. [1], on the basis of clinical observations and temporal bone studies, presented the hypothesis that endolymphatic hydrops can result from chronic otitis media. Saito et al. [2], on the basis of temporal bone studies, reported that 44.8% of ears with histological evidence of otitis media had a distended Reissner's membrane.

The above evidence suggested a close relationship between endolymphatic hydrops and otitis media, with the former possibly resulting from the spread of middle ear inflammation into the inner ear through the oval or round window.

This study was conducted in order to assess the possible relationship between endolymphatic hydrops and otitis media. The results of tests of endolymphatic hydrops and the occurrence of clinical symptoms related to endolymphatic hydrops in patients with chronic otitis media are described. Representative patients who appeared to have endolymphatic hydrops associated with chronic otitis media are also described.

Subjects and Methods

The subjects were 67 patients with chronic otitis media (30 males, 37 females), aged from 9–72 years, who underwent tympanoplasty or radical mastoidectomies at the Department of Otolaryngology of the Kobe City General Hospital from October, 1987 to November, 1988. All subjects underwent the glycerol test and electrocochleography (ECochG) before surgery, to test for endolymphatic hydrops. For comparison, another 34 ears were used (17 males, 17 females) in patients with Ménière's disease aged from 35–74 years.

After standard pure tone audiometry, glycerol (1.3 g/kg body weight) was orally administered for the glycerol test. After 3 h audiometry was performed again, and if the threshold of bone conduction was improved by more than 10 dB at more than 2 frequencies, the test was regarded as positive. ECochG was performed by an extratympanic technique, and a $-SP/AP$ amplitude ratio of more than 0.37 was regarded as positive.

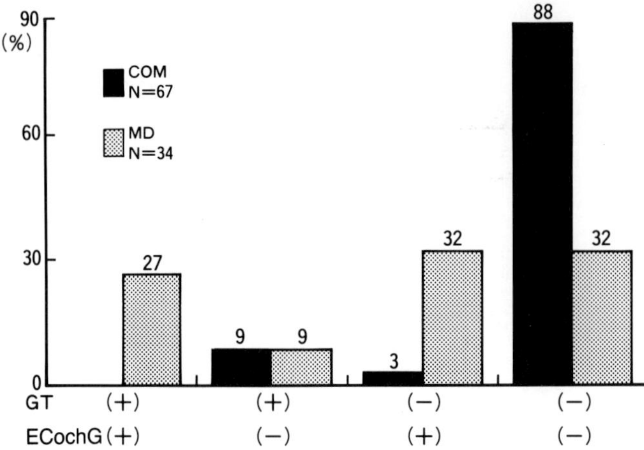

Fig. 25.1. Results of testing for endolymphatic hydrops test. COM, chronic otitis media; MD, Ménière's disease; GT, glycerol test, ECochG, electrocochleography

Results

Results of Testing for Endolymphatic Hydrops

The results of the glycerol test and ECochG were compared between the patients with chronic otitis media and those with Ménière's disease (Fig. 25.1). Among the 67 cases of chronic otitis media, no patient was positive for both tests. The glycerol test was positive and ECochG was negative in 6 ears (9%), the glycerol test was negative and ECochG was positive in 2 ears (3%), and both tests were negative in 59 ears (88%). In contrast, both tests were positive in 27% of the 34 patients with Ménière's disease. The glycerol test was positive and ECochG was negative in 9%, the glycerol test was negative and ECochG was positive in 32%, and both tests were negative in only 32%.

Clinical Features of Chronic Otitis Media Related to Endolymphatic Hydrops

It was judged that endolymphatic hydrops was present if either one of the 2 tests was positive. Among the 67 patients, it was judged that hydrops was present in 8 (12%) and absent in 59 (88%). In these 67 patients, the following clinical features were investigated.

Duration of Otitis Media

In patients with less than a 10-year history of disease, hydrops was present only in 6%, whereas it was found in 13% of those with a 10-20 year history, and in 20%

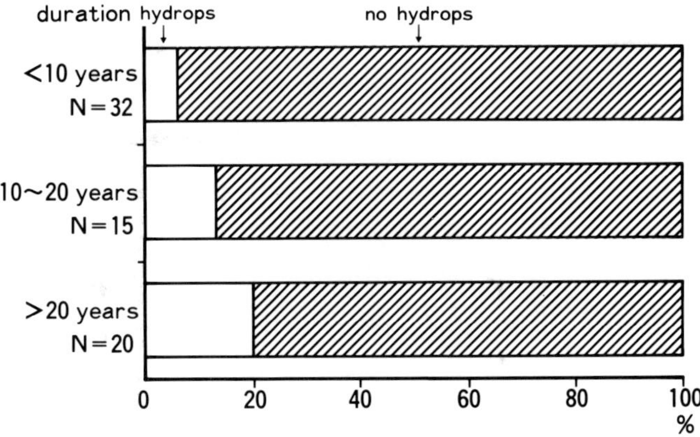

Fig. 25.2. Relationship between the duration of chronic otitis media and endolymphatic hydrops

of those with more than a 20-year history (Fig. 25.2). Thus, a longer duration of disease was associated with an increase in hydrops.

Presence of Vertigo

In patients with chronic otitis media and vertigo, hydrops was present in 30% of cases, but in chronic otitis media without vertigo it was seen only in 7% (Fig. 25.3). This difference was significant ($P < 0.01$).

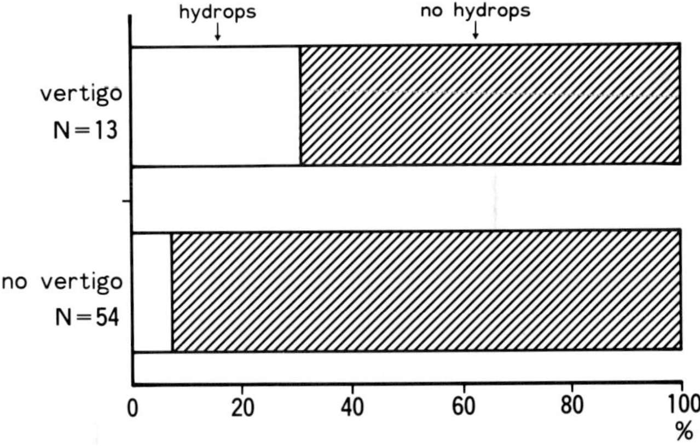

Fig. 25.3. Relationship between the presence of vertigo and endolymphatic hydrops

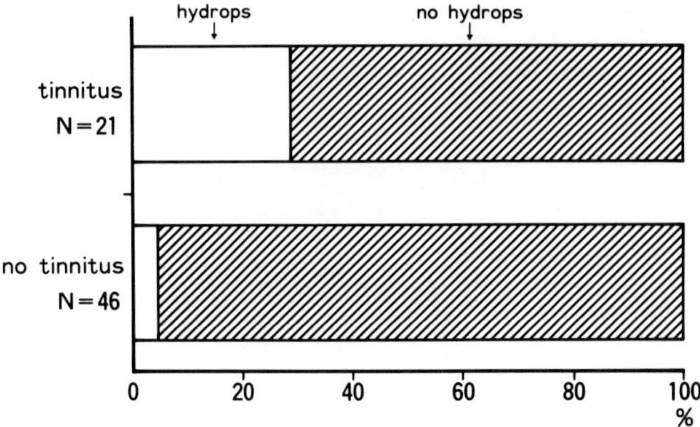

Fig. 25.4. Relationship between the presence of tinnitus and endolymphatic hydrops

Presence of Tinnitus

Hydrops was found in 29% of patients with chronic otitis media with tinnitus, but in chronic otitis media without tinnitus hydrops was only found in 4% (Fig. 25.4). Again, this difference was significant ($P < 0.05$).

Preoperative Bacteriological Testing of Ear Exudate

Hydrops was present in 24% of cases where bacteria were confirmed to be present in the ear exudate, but when bacteria were absent only 5% of cases had hydrops (Fig. 25.5). A tendency was noted for otitis media to be more active in patients with endolymphatic hydrops.

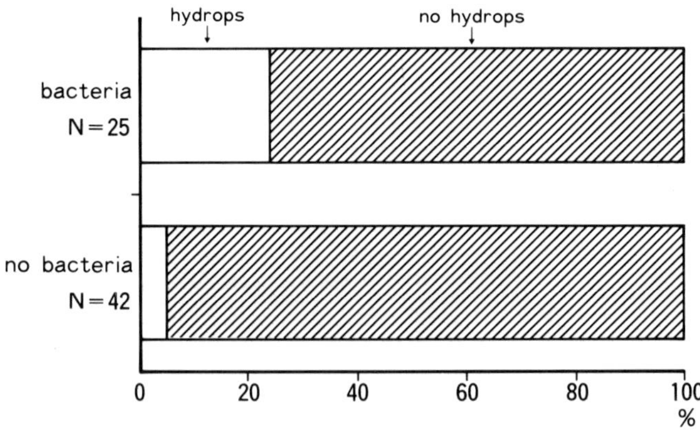

Fig. 25.5. Relationship between the presence of bacterial infection and endolymphatic hydrops

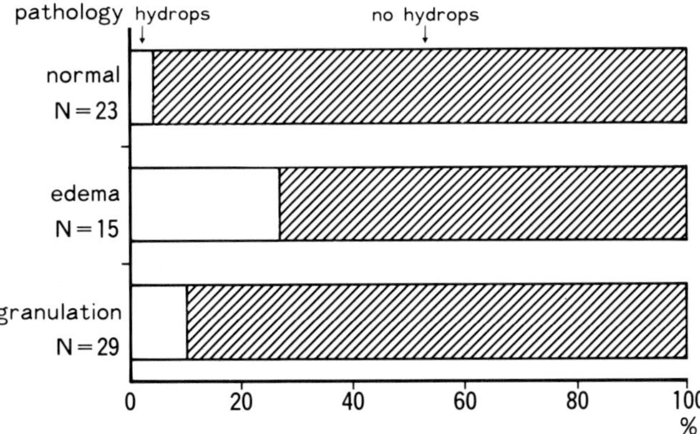

Fig. 25.6. Relationship between pathological changes of the oval window and endolymphatic hydrops

Pathological Changes in the Middle Ear Confirmed at the Time of Operation

The pathology in the middle ear, especially around the oval and round windows, were investigated and classified into normal, edema, or granulation. For the oval window (Fig. 25.6), endolymphatic hydrops was related to the presence of granulation and edema. For the round window as well (Fig. 25.7), it was noted that hydrops tended to be more common in patients with pathological changes. There was no significant difference between the rate of hydrops with regard to which window was affected.

Representative Cases

T. I. was a 47-year-old male who had a 40-year history of chronic suppurative otitis media in the left ear. He complained of progressive discharge and hearing loss

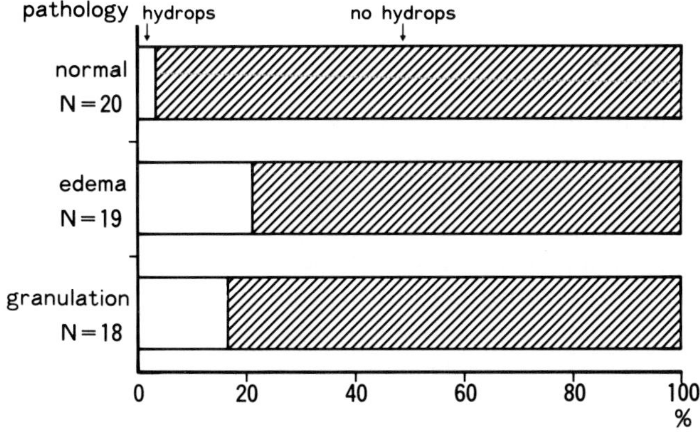

Fig. 25.7. Relationship between pathological changes of the round window and endolymphatic hydrops

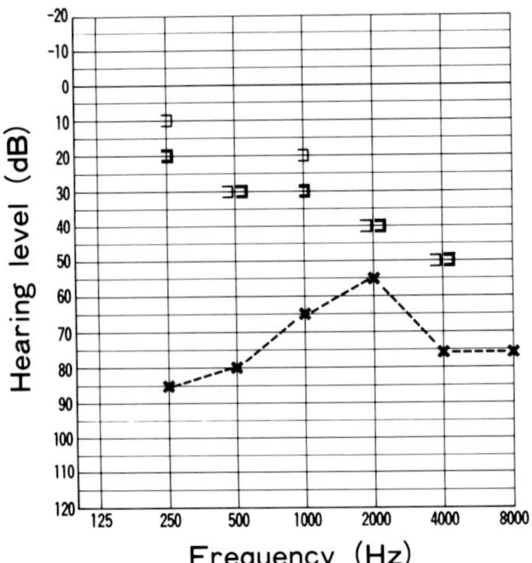

Fig. 25.8. Audiogram and preoperative glycerol test. Bone conduction before (⊐) and after (⊐) glycerol administration

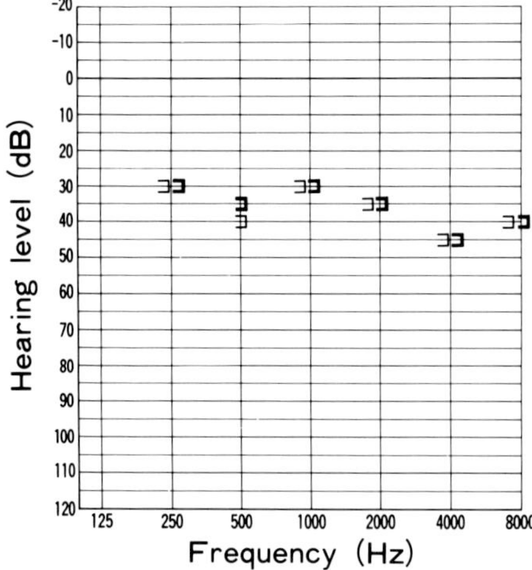

Fig. 25.9. Postoperative glycerol test. Bone conduction before (⊐) and after (⊐) glycerol administration

with continuous tinnitus in that ear for 8 months, and had repeated attacks of vertigo for 4 months. Pure tone audiometry of the left ear showed a mixed-type hearing loss and the glycerol test was positive (10 dB improvement of the threshold of bone conduction at 250 and 1000 Hz) (Fig. 25.8). The plain X-ray and the CT scan revealed a middle ear cholesteatoma, and an operation was performed. An attic cholesteatoma extending into the mastoid antrum and cavity and extensive granulation tissue contiguous with the round and oval windows were found at operation. The cholesteatoma and granulation tissue were completely removed and the first stage of the tympanoplasty procedure was performed. Ear discharge and vertigo disappeared after surgery, and the glycerol test was negative at the follow-up examination 2 months postoperatively (Fig. 25.9).

We also evaluated a 41-year-old female who had a positive preoperative and negative postoperative glycerol test.

Discussion

In Ménière's disease, the positive rate was 36% for the glycerol test and 59% for ECochG, while the rates in chronic otitis media were 9% and 3%, respectively. Endolymphatic hydrops was detected in 12% of chronic otitis media patients and in 68% of Ménière's disease patients, using the criterion that hydrops was present if either one of the two tests was positive. Thus, our study confirmed that endolymphatic hydrops can be present in chronic otitis media, although its incidence was lower than in Ménière's disease.

We presented a patient in whom a positive preoperative glycerol test became negative and whose vertigo disappeared after the treatment of pathological changes in the middle ear. Paparella et al. [1] and Saito [3] have also reported that vertigo disappeared or improved after surgery in patients with chronic otitis media and vertigo. These patients had endolymphatic hydrops induced by chronic otitis media. The temporal bone study by Saito et al. [2] showed that distension of Reissner's membrane was mild or moderate in otitis media. The above observations would suggest that endolymphatic hydrops caused by otitis media is a milder and more reversible condition than that seen in Ménière's disease.

We found that patients with chronic otitis media with a history of a long duration of illness, complaints of vertigo and tinnitus, and middle ear pathological changes (especially around the oval and round windows) developed endolymphatic hydrops more frequently. The pathways of the round and oval window are both possible as the route for middle ear pathology to spread to the inner ear. Although the main pathway is considered to be via the round window [4, 5], this could not be determined conclusively in this study because we found no significant difference in the degree of pathological changes between the round and oval windows in the patients with hydrops.

Surgical removal of middle ear disease is the definitive treatment of endolymphatic hydrops, but conservative treatment (steroids, isobide, antibiotics) [6] should be tried before surgery.

Conclusion

To assess the relationship between endolymphatic hydrops and otitis media, 34 patients with Ménière's disease and 67 patients with chronic otitis media underwent the glycerol test and ECochG. The clinical features of chronic otitis media related to the presence of endolymphatic hydrops were also investigated. Endolymphatic hydrops was detected in 12% of all cases of chronic otitis media and in 68% of those with Ménière's disease. Unlike that seen in Ménière's disease, this type of hydrops seemed to be milder and more reversible in nature. Chronic otitis media of long duration, vertigo, tinnitus, and pathological changes in the middle ear were associated with the more frequent occurrence of endolymphatic hydrops.

References

1. Paparella MM, Goycoolea MV, Meyerhoff WL, Shea D (1979) Endolymphatic hydrops and otitis media. Laryngoscope 89:43–58
2. Saito H, Kitahara M, Kitajima K, Takeda T, Yazawa D, Matsubara H, Kitano J (1981) Distended Reissner's membrane and otitis media (in Japanese). Pract Otol (Kyoto) 74: (Suppl 5) 2413–2418
3. Saito H (1982) Middle ear disease and vestibular function (in Japanese). Equilibrium Res 41:226–230
4. Goycoolea MV, Paparella MM, Juhn SK, Carpenter A-M (1980) Oval and round window changes in otitis media. Potential pathways between middle and inner ear. Laryngoscope 90:1387–1391
5. Paparella MM, Shea D, Meyerhoff WL, Goycoolea MV (1980) Silent otitis media. Laryngoscope 90:1089–1098
6. Isoda S, Kitahara M, Kitano T (1988) Treatment of endolymphatic hydrops caused by otitis media (in Japanese). Equilibrium Res [Suppl] 4:109–110

Chapter 26

Sudden Deafness with Bilateral Endolymphatic Hydrops

Mikio Suzuki and Masaaki Kitahara

There are numerous causes for deafness of sudden onset such as temporal bone fracture, viral labyrinthitis, otitic barotrauma, vestibular schwannoma, and Ménière's disease [1]. Since these causes often evade clear recognition, many cases of deafness of sudden onset are labeled as acute idiopathic auditory failure (sudden deafness). A significant number of these cases, however, are actually due to endolymphatic hydrops (EH).

In 1950, Williams et al. hypothesized that EH was the cause of sudden deafness in certain patients [2]; they also demonstrated that EH occasionally exists without vertigo, and that it characteristically leads to fluctuating hearing loss with a tendency toward greater damage to low tones than to high tones. Hallberg described certain cases of Ménière's syndrome in which sudden deafness was the first symptom [3]. At our clinic, 34 out of 80 (42%) patients with sudden deafness had confirmed EH [4]. These findings suggest that patients with fluctuating hearing loss attributable to EH may subsequently develop sudden deafness or Ménière's-type symptoms. Moreover, it is quite probable that patients with unilateral sudden deafness and bilateral EH will develop Ménière's-type symptoms or severe hearing loss in the ear contralateral to that with sudden deafness ("the contralateral ear"). This is a serious concern for cases of sudden deafness, since the contralateral ear is the only functional one they posses. The present report focuses on such cases of sudden deafness associated with bilateral fluctuating hearing loss attributable to EH.

Subjects

30 cases of sudden deafness were treated at our clinic in a two and a-half-year period from 1987 to 1989. Pure tone audiometry was performed at regular intervals on all patients throughout the course of treatment. In this study, fluctuating hearing loss was defined as a change in hearing level of 20 dB or more at two or more of the test frequencies of 250, 500, 1000, 2000, 4000 and 8000 Hz. Electrocochleography and dehydration tests (glycerol test, frosemid test) were used as a basis for judging whether fluctuating hearing loss was related to EH [5–7]. Of the 30 cases of sudden deafness, 13 displayed fluctuating hearing losses considered due to EH (43%); 4 had fluctuating hearing losses in both ears, 4 in the sudden deafness ear only, and

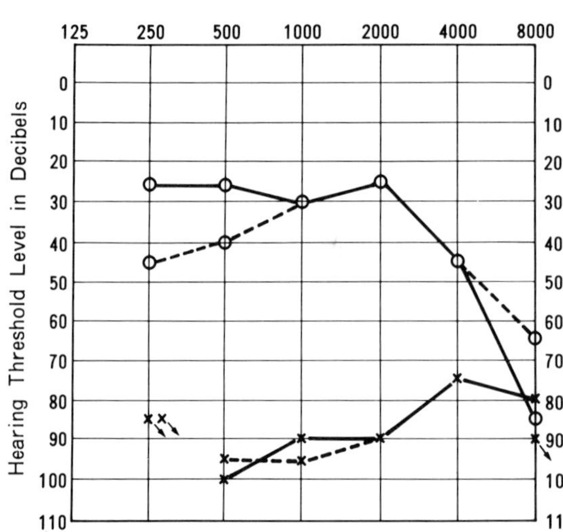

Fig. 26.1. Case 1: pure tone audiogram. *Solid line* shows the hearing threshold level at the onset of sudden deafness (Sept. 20, 1988). The *dotted line* shows the hearing threshold level when the patient was aware of hearing loss and tinnitus in the right ear (Nov. 2, 1988). o, right ear; ×, left ear. Masking used, band noise 60dB (250, 500, 1000, 2000 Hz)

5 only in the contralateral ear. The 4 patients with fluctuating hearing losses in both ears were the subjects of the present study.

Case Reports

Case 1

The patient, a 46-year-old Oriental male with no previous history of otological symptoms, experienced sudden hearing loss and tinnitus in his left ear on September 19 1988. He was unaware of any otological symptoms in his right ear. The day following an episode of dizziness he consulted an otolaryngologist. Pure tone audiometry revealed profound sensorineural hearing loss in his left ear and a high frequency hearing loss of unknown origin in the right ear (Fig. 26.1). He was started on a program of treatment including medications such as predonisolone (30 mg for 3 days), vitamin B_{12}, and adenosine-triphosphate. Two weeks later he was referred to our clinic due to continued hearing loss and tinnitus in his left ear. The glycerol test was positive in the left ear, and dominant negative summating potentials (DNSP) were observed in the electrocochleograms (ECochGs) of both ears. Other audiological examinations (speech audiometry, SISI test, Bekesy audiometry, and tympanometry) indicated that hearing loss in the left ear was of the cochlear type. There was a weak caloric response to ice water in both ears. The VDRL and TPHA tests were negative. The glucose tolerance test was normal. X-ray temporal bone and computed tomography of the brain revealed no abnormalities. Bilateral EH was presumed in light of the examination results.

The course of the patient's pure tone audiometry is shown in Fig. 26.2. Profound fluctuating hearing loss and tinnitus in the left ear showed no improvement in spite of a course of steroid therapy (hydrocortisone 600 mg, 300 mg, 100 mg each for three days). The patient experienced the first episode of vertigo (lasting about 5

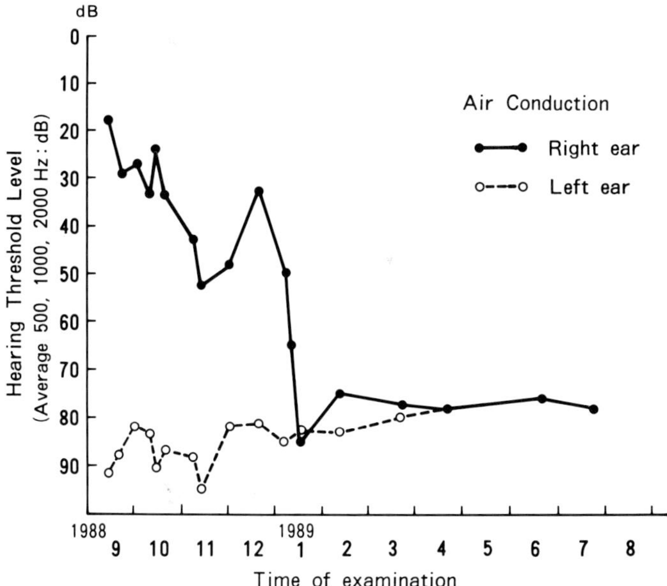

Fig. 26.2. Case 1: hearing threshold level throughout the course of treatment. The *solid line* represents the level in the right ear and the *dotted line*, that in the left ear

minutes) with no worsening of tinnitus and hearing loss on October 9 1988. Subsequent dizziness occurred several times a week for 3 weeks. He was unaware of hearing loss or tinnitus in the right ear although fluctuating of hearing levels in both ears were revealed by pure tone audiometry from the onset of the sudden deafness in the left ear. He noted a slight loss of hearing and tinnitus in the right ear on November 2 1988 (Fig. 26.1). Fluctuations in hearing in the right ear continued, but overall hearing levels gradually worsened despite the administration of an oral steroid agent (betamethasone 1.5 mg/day for one week). Speech discrimination was 50% in the right ear and 5% in the left ear. The patient was hospitalized and received a second course of steroid therapy. Hearing in both ears showed a gradual improvement, but no change was reported in the patient's tinnitus. Hearing levels had recovered to an averaged level of 35 dB in the right ear and 82 dB in the left ear by December 16 1988.

Renewed hearing loss accompanied by a 10-min episode of dizziness in the right ear occurred on January 9 1989. Hearing levels averaged 90 dB in the right ear and 87 dB in the left ear on January 17 1989. The patient was rehospitalized and received a third course of steroid therapy. A slight improvement has occurred in the hearing of his right ear, but in general his bilateral hearing loss has remained profound.

Case 2

The patient, a 47-year-old Oriental male with a 10-year history of bilateral tinnitus, experienced sudden hearing loss and increased tinnitus in his left ear with accompanying dizziness on September 11 1988. He was treated at our clinic on the following

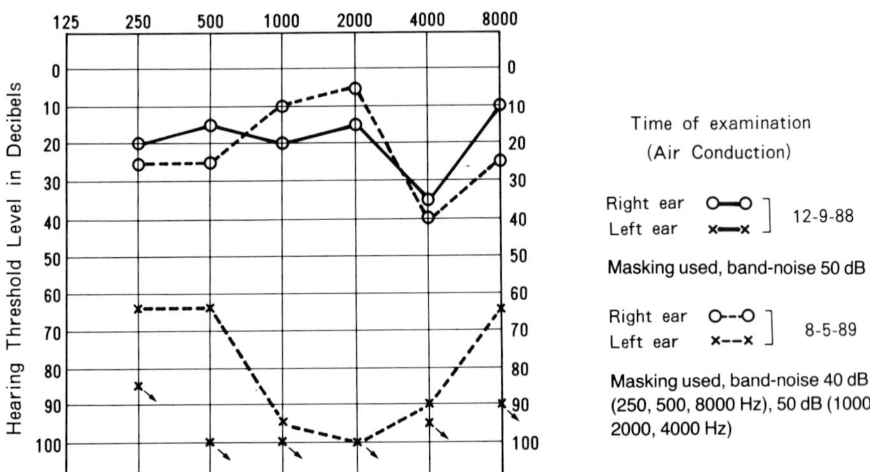

Fig. 26.3. Case 2: pure tone audiogram. *Solid line* shows the hearing threshold level at the onset of sudden deafness (Sept. 20, 1988). The *dotted line* shows the hearing threshold level when the patient felt fullness in the right ear (May 8, 1989). o, right ear; ×, left ear

day. Pure tone audiometry revealed total deafness on the left and slight sensorineural loss characterized by a c5 dip pattern on the right (Fig. 26.3). The history for noise exposure was positive, but he had never noted hearing loss or experienced vertigo. He had hypertrophic obstructive cardiomyopathy successfully controlled through the use of a β-blocker.

The glycerol test was negative in both ears and a DNSP was observed in the ECochG of his right ear. Both ears showed a decreased caloric response. Other audiological examinations revealed that the hearing loss in the left ear was of the cochlear type. The VDRL and TPHA tests were negative and fasting blood glucose was normal. X-ray temporal bone and computed tomography of the brain revealed no abnormalities. He was unaware of hearing loss in the right ear although fluctuation of hearing level was detected by pure tone audiometry from the onset of the sudden hearing loss (Fig. 26.4). Fluctuation of hearing level in the left ear, of which he was also unaware, had started on Oct. 1988 (Fig. 26.4) The examinations described above indicate EH to be the cause of the fluctuating hearing loss. The patient reported a feeling of fullness in the right ear in April 1989 (Fig. 26.3).

Case 3

The patient, a 46-year-old Oriental female, experienced sudden hearing loss and tinnitus in her left ear accompanied by episodic vertigo on April 25 1988. An examination by an otolaryngologist revealed profound hearing loss in her left ear; her right ear was unremarkable. Treatment, primarily with steroids, resulted in only

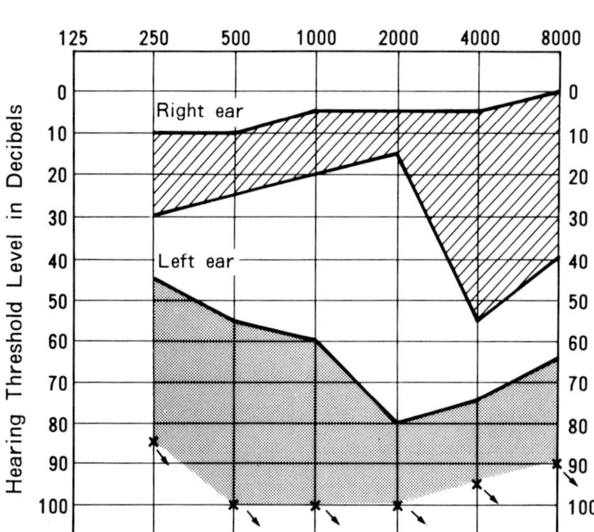

Fig. 26.4. Case 2: fluctuation of hearing level in both ears throughout the course of treatment (Sept. '88–July '89)

minor improvement, so she was referred to our clinic on June 13 1988. Pure tone audiometry revealed a profound hearing loss in the left ear and a mild hearing loss in the right ear (Fig. 26.5).

The glycerol test was negative in both ears and a DNSP was observed in the ECochG of the right ear. There was a decreased caloric response in the left ear. The VDRL and TPHA tests were negative and fasting blood glucose was normal. X-ray temporal bone and computed tomography of the brain revealed no abnormalities.

From May 1989, the patient noted a slight hearing loss and fullness in her right ear; testing revealed bilateral fluctuating hearing loss (Fig. 26. 6). Pure tone audiometry revealed a low-frequency sensorineural hearing loss on the right (Fig. 26.5).

Case 4

The patient, a 54-year-old Oriental female, experienced sudden hearing loss and fullness in her left ear on December 6 1988. She had no cochlear symptoms in her right ear. She reported slight unsteadiness on December 12 1988, and was hospitalized on December 13. Pure tone audiometry revealed a profound hearing loss in the left ear and a mild low frequency together with a moderate high frequency sensorineural hearing loss in the right ear (Fig. 26.7). Impedence audiometry showed normal compliance.

The glycerol test was positive on the left and negative on the right. A DNSP was seen in the ECochG of the right ear. There was a normal caloric response in each

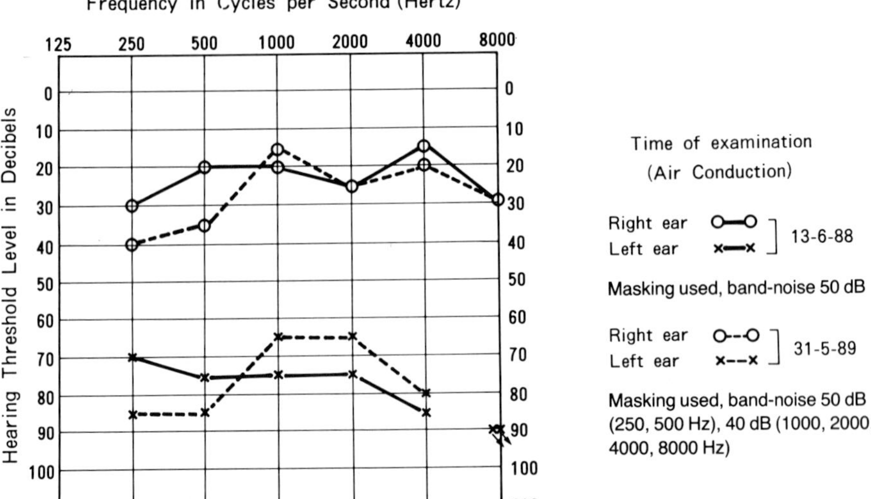

Fig. 26.5. Case 3: pure tone audiogram. *Solid line* shows the hearing threshold level 2 months after the onset of sudden deafness (June 13, 1988). The *dotted line* shows the hearing threshold level when the patient detected hearing loss in the right ear (May 31, 1989), o, right ear; ×, left ear

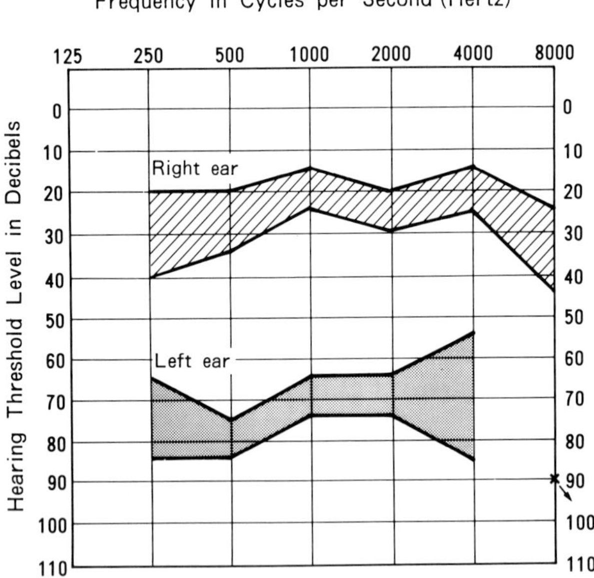

Fig. 26.6. Case 3: fluctuation of hearing level in both ears throughout the course of treatment (June '88–July '89)

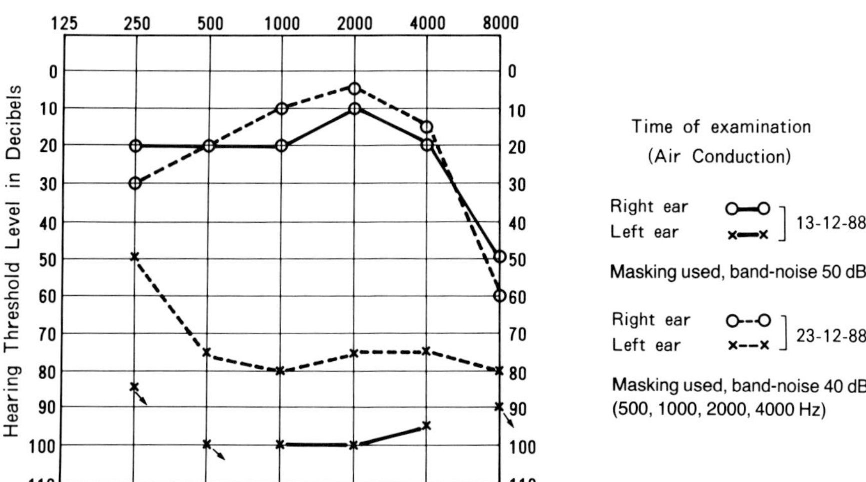

Fig. 26.7. Case 4: pure tone audiogram: *Solid line* shows the hearing threshold level at the onset of sudden deafness (Dec. 13, 1988). The *dotted line* shows the hearing threshold level when the patient felt fullness in the right ear (Dec. 23, 1988). o, right ear; ×, left ear

ear. The VDRL and TPHA tests were negative, while the glucose tolerance test revealed a diabetic condition. X-ray temporal bone and computerized tomography of the brain showed no abnormalities. These findings indicated EH in both ears.

Although fluctuating hearing loss in both ears were revealed by pure tone audiometry from the time of onset of sudden deafness, she was unaware of hearing loss in her right ear (Fig. 26.8). The patient received a course of steroid therapy combined with subcutaneous injections of insulin. Hearing in the left ear improved, but failed to attain normal levels. She had noted fullness in her right ear from December 20 1988 (Fig. 26.7). The administration of a diuretic (isosorbide) resulted in a one-month disappearance of the sensation of fullness. Nevertheless, bilateral fluctuating hearing loss have persisted.

The data on the above 4 patients with bilateral EH are summarized in Table 26.1. Fluctuating hearing loss in the contralateral ear were verified by audiometry at the onset of sudden deafness in cases 1, 2, and 4, and 13 months later in case 3, although the patients themselves became aware of otological symptoms (hearing loss, tinnitus, fullness, etc.) in the contralateral ear only after a period of from 0.5 month–13 months following the attacks of sudden deafness. Two of the patients had decreased caloric test responses in both ears, and one in the suddenly deaf ear only. These caloric test responses were similar to those of the contralateral type of delayed endolymphatic hydrops. The patients received one or more courses of steroid therapy (hydrocortisone 600 mg, 300 mg, and 100 mg for three days, respectively), and hearing levels are now being monitored in an effort to prevent future severe hearing loss.

Table 26.1. Sudden deafness associated with bilateral endolymphatic hydrops.

Patient	Sudden hearing loss	Age	Time span between sudden deafness and awareness of contralateral ear symptoms (Months)	ECochG		Glycerol test		Calorics	
				R	L	R	L	R	L
1	L	46	1.5	P	N	UC	P	DVR	DVR
2	L	47	7	P	—	N	N	DVR	DVR
3	L	46	13	P	—	N	N	N	DVR
4	L	54	0.5	N	—	UC	P	N	N

R, right; L, Left; P, positive; UC, unclear; N, negative (ECochG, glycerol test), normal (Calorics); DVR, decreased vestibular response; — not measurable

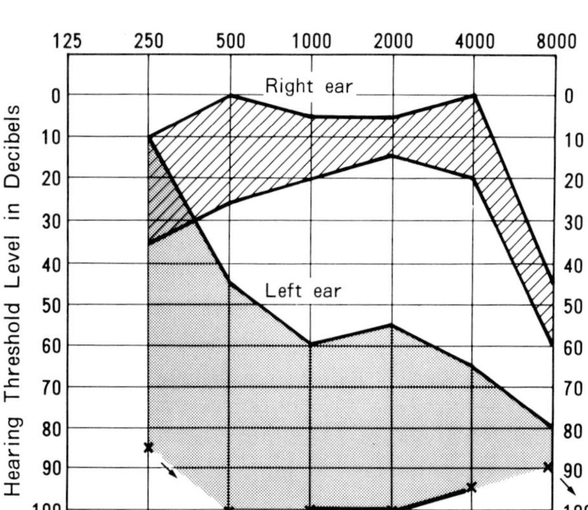

Fig. 26.8. Case 4: fluctuation of hearing level in both ears throughout the course of treatment (Dec. '88–March '89)

Discussion

Some patients who present with sudden deafness eventually develop the symptoms of Ménière's syndrome. Williams suggested that certain cases of sudden deafness might be attributable to EH [2]. Hallberg reported that the initial symptom in 56 of the 1270 patients he treated with Ménière's syndrome was sudden deafness [3]. This evidence indicates that fluctuating hearing loss considered to be due to EH may lead to sudden deafness. Experience at our clinic verifies this: 42% of the patients with sudden deafness had EH in the affected ears [4]. If the contralateral ear has a fluctuating hearing loss associated with EH, there is a high probability that severe hearing loss will eventually occur in this ear.

The etiology of sudden deafness is often unclear. The most spectacular and consistent pathological changes are atrophy of the organ of Corti, the stria vascularis, and the tectorial membrane [1]. Cases of sudden deafness have also been seen in association with EH [8, 9] and rupture of Reissner's membrane [10]. Lawrence and McCabe [11] suggested that rupture and rehealing of Reissner's membrane may underlie the episodic nature of Ménière's disease. Schuknecht [12] has made similar observations on several occasions. The occurrence of such injury in the contralateral ear as well indicates that even in the absence of severe hearing loss there is a high likelihood of the development of EH.

In this paper a case was presented in which sudden deafness occurred in an ear with previously existing fluctuating hearing loss attributable to EH (the right ear in Case 1). The same pattern may have been present in the remaining cases as well, but this was impossible to verify since the patients were observed only subsequent to their presenting with sudden deafness. Patients with bilateral EH are often unaware that a fluctuating hearing loss exists in both ears until the hearing loss is severe: audiometic evaluations of 3 out of 4 cases described above revealed fluctuating hearing loss in the contralateral ears at the onset of sudden deafness, yet the patients remained unaware of such losses for a considerable period of time making it easy to overlook the fluctuation of hearing levels in the contralateral ear. Hearing levels in both ears must be monitored carefully.

Schuknecht [13] studied the clinical manifestations of 18 cases of delayed endolymphatic hydrops. This condition is divided into ipsilateral and contralateral types. The criteria for classification as ipsilateral delayed endolymphatic hydrops are: 1) profound hearing loss in one or both ears discovered incidentally in childhood or related to some specific disease or trauma, and 2) subsequent onset of episodic vertigo of the Ménière's type. The criteria for classification as contralateral delayed endolymphatic hydrops are: 1) profound hearing loss in one ear, discovered incidentally in childhood or related to some specific disease or trauma, and 2) subsequent onset in the opposite ear of fluctuating hearing loss, with or without episodic vertigo of the Ménière's type. Schuknecht attributed these clinical symptoms to endolymphatic hydrops resulting from a slow—often over a period of many years—accumulation of endolymph. He described 4 of 22 ipsilateral cases and 2 of 21 contralateral cases which had early histories of sudden deafness [14]. In the present study, 3 of the 4 cases presented had fluctuating hearing losses in both the suddenly deaf ears and in the contralateral ears monitored from the onset of sudden deafness. This suggests that EH is present in many patients earlier than Schuknecht had estimated in his study. There is a strong likelihood that delayed endolymphatic hydrops includes certain cases of sudden deafness associated with bilateral EH, a possibility which we are presently investigating through EH testing at the onset of sudden deafness.

Bilateral EH in association with unilateral sudden deafness has the potential for causing subsequent severe hearing loss in both ears. Of the 30 patients with sudden deafness examined in the present study, 4 cases with this condition were found, in addition to 5 cases which had fluctuating hearing losses considered to be due to EH in the contralateral ear only. Hence 9 out of 30 cases of sudden deafness (30%) were potential examples of this condition. It is thus important to check for EH in both ears at the onset of sudden deafness, even if a patient does not complain of hearing loss, tinnitus, and fullness in the contralateral ear. An early diagnosis of EH, particularly in the contralateral ear, will provide a more accurate prognosis of the patient's hearing levels and can help prevent severe bilateral hearing loss in the future.

We have assigned the term "sudden deafness with bilateral endolymphatic hydrops" to cases of acute sensorineural hearing loss associated with bilateral fluctuating hearing loss attributable to EH. This condition deserves greater attention, since patients with this condition could develop severe bilateral hearing loss in the future.

Summary

The clinical findings on 4 cases of sudden deafness with bilateral fluctuating hearing loss attributable to EH suggest that endolymphatic hydrops has the potential for causing future hearing impairments. Depending upon the case, the time of appearance of the clinical symptoms in the two ears can vary significantly. Monitoring the hearing levels in both ears may enable the minimization of hearing loss in the ear contralateral to the initially affected side.

References

1. Schuknecht HF, Kimura RS, Naufal PM (1973) The pathology of sudden deafness. Acta Otolaryngol (Stockh) 76:75–97
2. Williams HL, Horton BT, Day LA (1950) Endolymphatic hydrops without vertigo. Arch Otolaryngol 51:557–581
3. Hallberg OE (1956) Sudden deafness of obscure origin. Laryngoscope 66:1237–1267
4. Schu S, Kitano H, Isoda K, Ozawa H, Izukura H (1986) Sudden deafness and endolymphatic hydrops (in Japanese). J Otolaryngol Jpn 89:525
5. Kitahara M, Takeda T, Yazawa Y, Matsubara H (1981) Electrocochleography in the diagnosis of Ménière's disease. In: Vosteen K-H, Schuknecht HF, Pfaltz CR, Wersäll J, Kimura RS, Morgenstern C, Juhn SK (eds) Ménière's disease: Pathogenesis, diagnosis and treatment. Thieme-Stratton, New York, p 163
6. Klockhoff I, Lindblom U (1967) Glycerol test in Ménière's disease. Acta Otolaryngol [Suppl] (Stockh) 224:450–451
7. Matsubara H, Kitahara M, Takeda T, Yazawa Y (1985) Rebound phenomenon in glycerol test. Acta Otolaryngol [Suppl] (Stockh) 419:115–122
8. Karmody CS (1983) Viral labyrinthitis: early pathology in the human. Laryngoscope 93:1527–1533
9. Sando I, Harada T, Loehr A, Sobel JH (1977) Sudden deafness. Ann Otol Rhinol Laryngol 86:269–279
10. Gussen R (1983) Sudden deafness associated with bilateral Reissner's membrane ruptures. Am J Otol 4:27–32
11. Lawrence M, McCabe BF (1959) Inner ear mechanics and deafness. JAMA 171:1927–1932
12. Schuknecht HF (1963) Ménière's disease: A correlation of symptomatology and pathology. Laryngoscope 73:651–665
13. Schuknecht HF (1978) Delayed endolymphatic hydrops. Ann Otol Rhinol Laryngol 87:743–748
14. Schuknecht HF (1985) Neurolabyrinthitis: viral infections of the peripheral auditory and vestibular system. In: Nomura Y (ed) Hearing loss and dizziness, 1st edn. Igaku-Shoin, Tokyo

Chapter 27

Secondary or Idiopathic Endolymphatic Hydrops?

Masaaki Kitahara and Yoshiro Yazawa

It is widely accepted that Ménière's is an idiopathic disease involving the membranous inner ear. Disease which cause secondary endolymphatic hydrops (SEH) are differentiated from Ménière's disease. Theoretically this idea is acceptable, but it is quite difficult to distinguish SEH from idiopathic endolymphatic hydrops (IEH). In other words, when symptoms similar to those of Ménière's disease coexist with another definitive disease, we find difficulty in determining whether the symptoms are caused by the disease itself or whether they are truly those of Ménière's disease. In this paper, we will discuss this controversial problem in diagnosing Ménière's disease.

Diseases Which Cause Ménière's-like Symptoms and Those Which Do Not

If the term Ménière's syndrome (disease) were used in cases where their etiology is both known and unknown (A. J. Duval III, Per-G Lundquist, see chap. 1), we would never be faced with this difficult problem. However, most researchers do not accept this viewpoint. The authors made an international survey of ideas on what diseases are considered to be causes of Ménière's symptoms and those which are not. Jongkees [1] writes that "Ménière's disease is an idiopathic syndrome; if the clinical picture is complicated by either otitis, otosclerosis, mumps, high blood pressure, diabetes, syphilis etc., it is not wise to call these probably secondary reactions to a primary ailment, Ménière's disease. The diagnosis is already a tricky one. If we want to treat (patients suffering from) Ménière's disease, let us use the right words in the right place. In complicated cases, treat the underlying disease, not the secondary Ménière's syndrome." He also writes in another paper [2] that the difficulty with the name Ménière's is that it covers two concepts—Ménière's disease and Ménière's syndrome—which should be carefully kept apart. Quoting Wilmot's paper [3] Jongkees states that Ménière's disease is a rather rare disease. Wilmot [3] writes that Ménière's disease must satisfy several positive and negative criteria. Some criteria are: (1) the tympanic membranes, middle ears, and conducting hearing mechanisms are normal on both sides, (2) eustachian tube function in both ears is normal, and (3) There is no history of chronic ill-health and no evidence of such on clinical examination. G. Zechner (1980, personal communication) also states that Ménière's disease includes the idiopathic form and excludes all Ménière's-like symptoms in cases of diabetes, cervical spine syndrome, hypotension, hypertension, metabolic disease, nephritis, and so on. These researchers are considered to be representative of those who insist upon excluding Ménière's disease when other already known and extremely varied diseases are present. Their real intention in extensively excluding Ménière's disease from their cases is suggested by the following two points. The first is to give special warning lest one should be led on the wrong diagnostic path, since a great many doctors do not have the necessary knowledge, experience, and clinical sensitivity to separate the true from the false Ménière's patient (L. B. W. Jongkees 1980, personal communication). The second is to have comparable cases to work with and to analyze genuine research work or in performing drug trials (T. J. Wilmot 1980, personal communication). Wilmot, of course, realizes that Ménière's disease and other conditions can co-exist independently. But he just didn't want to evaluate Ménière's disease coexisting with other conditions, in terms of his auditory and vestibular analysis techniques, as cases of pure Ménière's disease. These rigid criteria seem to be used not for clinical but for special purposes.

It is generally understood that two or more diseases can co-exist in a person. Ménière's disease should not be the exception to the above concensus. B. McCabe (1980, personal communication) states that there is no question that Ménière's disease can co-exist with other diseases such as hypertension and brain tumor, and other ear diseases for that matter. Otosclerosis would be the most likely co-existing ear disease in the event of two diagnoses, just as he would be diagnosed as having essential hypertension and tuberculosis if he had both of these affections. M.G. Graham (1980, personal communication) feels that the underlying conditions or diseases with Ménière's-type symptoms are specific ones, such as lues, hypothyroidism, diabetes. These have been described as having a close relationship with Ménière's disease. He thinks that one can decide whether or not the underlying diseases is related to the symptoms by treating it. As is demonstrated in lues and diabetes, symptoms will often improve with respective treatments of the disease. According to H. O. Barber (1980, personal communication), SEH is caused by such known conditions as syphilis, serous labyrinthitis, labyrinthitis ossificans, temporal bone fracture, and acoustic neuroma. However, other diseases, such as brain tumor, hypertension, etc., may co-exist with Ménière's disease and nearly always it would be by chance, and not by causal association. R. Hinchcliffe (1980, personal communication) states that since a person may have not one but several diseases, other conditions may co-exist with Ménière's disease. Thus one should not exclude a diagnosis of Ménière's disease merely because the person has some other condition—unless that condition, like syphilis, or periarteritis nodosa, precludes that the aural condition is something other than Ménière's disease (e.g., late congenital syphilis or Cogan's syndrome respectively). He also states that to argue that the endolymphatic hydrops (EH) must be idiopathic would exclude cases where there has been microscopic evidence for some anomaly of the internal ear structures. He thinks this would be wrong. One would expect that more careful searching of the structures of internal ears affected by EH would provide increasing evidence for some structural abnormality (congenital or acquired). His problem, and also that of many others, is that if one accepts that Ménière's disease is a psychosomatic one, why should it be located in one particular organ of the body and on one side only, as indeed it usually is? This localization is accounted for under psychosomatic concepts as being due to the locus minoris resistentiae—in other words, that we have a "weak organ." The "weak organ" concept implies that there is some structural inadequacy of the involved organ. J.D.L. Smyth (1980, personal communication) agrees that other conditions can co-exist independently with Ménière's disease and that they are probably often contributory to the underlying problem but not necessarily responsible for the onset of Ménière's disease. K. Janke (1980, personal communication) does not believe that brain tumors or hypertension may cause Ménière's-type symptoms but accepts that they may co-exist occasionally. He thinks, however, that in Ménière's disease a predisposition of the inner ear becomes clinically manifest by a trigger, e.g., allergic, metabolic, toxic or autonomic imbalance.

The following are diseases which are thought to cause the development of SEH: congenital syphilis, syphilis, leukemia, Paget's disease, delayed hydrops, otosclerosis, carcinoma of the ear, subacute labyrinthitis, temporal bone fracture, acoustic neurinoma, hypoglycemia, hyper- and hypotension, multiple sclerosis, basilar insufficiency, Wallenberg's syndrome. When these diseases are diagnosed in cases with symptoms similar to those in Ménière's disease, the diagnoses exclude Ménière's disease. Whereas otosclerosis, brain tumor, hypertension, basilar insufficiency, and all other diseases excluding congenital syphilis and Cogan's syndrome are diseases which are recognized as not being responsible for the development of EH. These diseases are thought to be able to co-exist independently with Ménière's disease. In other words, these diseases are recognized as not having been responsible for the development of EH. These groups of diseases were compiled as a result of the international survey. It should be noted that the same diseases appear repeatedly in both groups. Though researchers generally believe that various kinds of diseases could independently co-exist with Ménière's disease, these diseases vary according to researchers.

Histopathological Findings of the Labyrinth in Cases Other Than Ménière's Disease

Table 27.1 shows histopathological findings of the labyrinth in cases of dizziness unrelated to Ménière's disease hitherto reported. This table also includes diseases other than Ménière's which showed distention of Reissner's membrane. In these diseases, various kinds of histological findings are observed in the labyrinth, in addition to the distention of Reissner's membrane. In labyrinthitis, ossification is observed in the scala tympani and rarely in the scala vestibuli at the basal turn of the cochlea. In congenital syphilis, absorbed bone is replaced by connective tissue and an infiltration of round cells is found. In Cogan's syndrome, ossification at the basal turn of the cochlea is observed. Each of these findings, however, is not present in all of the reported cases of the same disease. Therefore, it is not always possible

Table 27.1. Reported histopathological findings of temporal bones in cases of dizziness other than that related to Ménière's disease [4–37].

Disease	No of cases reported	
	Hydrops	Normal or collapse
Labyrinthitis	15(8) [4–7]	1 [4]
Congenital syphilis	5 (4) [8–10]	
Syphilis	1 (1) [11]	
Cogan's syndrome	2 (2) [12, 13]	
Otosclerosis	7 (2) [14–16]	2 [17, 15]
Leukemia	2 [18, 19]	2 [20, 21]
Sudden deafness	1 [19]	7 [19, 22–24]
Paget's disease	1 [25]	1 [26]
Sensory-neural deafness	3 [27, 28]	
Acoustic neurinoma and other CP angle tumors	3 [29, 30]	3 [30, 31, 24]
Temporal bone fracture	1 [32]	4 [32]
Congenital anomalies	4 (2) [33–36]	1 [37]

Numbers in paretheses indicate cases of bilateral hydrops.
Hydrops, cases with EH; Normal or Collapse, cases with normal labyrinth or endolymphatic collapse

to distinguish primary and SEH even by post-mortem histopathological examination of the labyrinth. However, if extension of Reissner's membrane is frequently observed in autopsy cases with specific diseases, then EH can be considered to be secondary to these diseases. Keeping in mind the above considerations, the findings in Table 1 reveal that Cogan's syndrome, labyrinthitis, and congenital syphilis develop EH at an extremely high incidence (100%, 90% and 100% respectively). The extent of distention of Reissner's membrane is severe in Paget's disease, acoustic neurinoma and congenital anomaly, while it is mild or moderate in cases of otosclerosis, leukemia, sudden deafness, and temporal bone fracture.

When we take a general view of both the results of the international survey and a review of the literature on autopsy findings, it is apparent that most of the researchers agree upon recognizing that EH is not primary but secondary when basic diseases such as labyrinthitis, Cogan's syndrome and congenital syphilis reveal—with high incidence—distention of Reissner's membrane at autopsy. When other diseases such as otosclerosis, temporal bone fracture, congenital anomaly etc., co-exist with symptoms similar to Ménière's disease, the idea as to whether the symptoms are due to Ménière's disease or not—i.e. is EH primary or secondary—differs according to the researchers. The Ménière's Disease Research Committee (1974) proposed that two or more diagnoses for a patient be made where it cannot be decided whether the inner ear pathology is primary or secondary.

In general when two or more pathologies co-exist in a person, treatments for these pathologies are necessary regardless of the fact that one may be the cause of the other. In cases of EH, this concept should also be applied irrespective of whether it is primary or secondary. In our practice, we have been successful with intramastoid drainage surgery for delayed hydrops and a combined treatment of steroids, isosorbide and tympanoplasty for SEH due to otitis media. If any new technique for the treatment of EH is obtained through the study of Ménière's disease, we must actively apply this technique to cases with probable SEH as well, in addition to giving the proper treatment for the co-existent diseases.

Summary

When specific diseases such as labyrinthitis, congenital syphilis and Cogan's disease are found in cases with symptoms similar to Ménière's disease, the symptoms are considered to be due to the specific diseases. When other disease such as otosclerosis, brain tumor etc. co-exist with similar symptoms to Ménière's disease, agreements have not been obtained whether the above diseases are the causes of the symptoms or not.

It was emphasized that treatment for both the disease and the endolymphatic pathology must be actively carried out in any event.

References

1. Jongkees LBW (1979) Some remarks on Ménière's disease. ORL J Otorhinolaryngol Relat Spec 42: 1–5
2. Jongkees LBW (1975) Vertigo. J Vertigo 1: 1–7
3. Wilmot TJ (1974) Vestibular analysis in Ménière's disease. J Laryngol Otol 88: 295–306
4. Paparella MM (1967) The pathology of suppurative labyrinthitis. Ann Otol Rhinol Laryngol 76: 554–586
5. Schuknecht HF (1976) Pathophysiology of endolymphatic hydrops. Arch Otorhinolaryngol 212: 253–262
6. Suga F, Lindsay JR (1977) Labyrinthitis ossificans. Ann Otol Rhinol Laryngol 86: 17–29
7. Hinojosa R, Lindsay JR (1980) Profound deafness. Arch Otolaryngol 106: 193–209
8. Karmody CS, Schuknecht HF (1966) Deafness in congenital syphilis. Arch Otolaryngol 83: 18–27
9. Schuknecht HF (1974) Pathology of the ear. Harvard University Press, Cambridge
10. Belal A Jr (1980) Dandy's syndrome. Am J Otol 1: 151–156
11. Linthicum FH, El-Rahman AGB (1987) Hydrops due to syphilitic endolymphatic duct obliteration. Laryngoscope 97: 568–574
12. Wolff D (1965) The pathology of Cogan's syndrome causing profound deafness. Ann Otol Rhinol Laryngol 74: 507–520
13. Zechner G (1980) Zum Cogan-Syndrom. Acta Otolaryngol (Stockh) 89: 310–316
14. Johnsson LG, Hawkins JE, Linthicum FH (1978) Cochlear and vestibular lesions in capsular otosclerosis as seen in microdissection. Ann Otol Rhinol Laryngol 87 (Suppl 48): 1–40
15. Liston SL, Paparella MM (1984) Otosclerosis and endolymphatic hydrops. Laryngoscope 94: 1003–1007
16. Schuknecht HF, Richer E (1980) Apical lesions of the cochlea in idiopathic endolymphatic hydrops and other disorders. ORL J Otorhinolaryngol Relat Spec 42: 46–76
17. Benitez JT, Schuknecht HF (1962) Otosclerosis. Laryngoscope 72: 1–9
18. Paparella MM (1973) Otological manifestations of leukemia. Laryngoscope 83: 1510–1526

19. Sando I, Egami T (1977) Inner ear hemorrhage and endolymphatic hydrops in a leukemic patient with sudden hearing loss. Ann Otol Rhinol Laryngol 86:518–524
20. Hallpike CS, Harrison MS (1950) Clinical and pathological observations on a case of leukemia with deafness and vertigo. J Laryngol Otol 64:427
21. La Venuta F (1972) Involvement of the inner ear in acute stem cell leukemia. Ann Otol Rhinol Laryngol 81:132–136
22. Takahara S (1972) Idiopathic endolymphatic hydrops with sudden onset of deafness (in Japanese). J Otolaryngol Jpn 77:959–969
23. Takahara S (1974) Pathology of temporal bone of the late Professor F. Tanaka (in Japanese). J Otolaryngol Jpn 77:805–906
24. Toriyama Y (1974) Histopathological findings in cases of sudden deafness (in Japanese). J Otolaryngol Jpn 46:827–835
25. Brunner H (1984) Ménière's disease. J Laryngol Otol 63:627–638
26. Brunner H (1936) Zur Kenntnis der Otitis deformans der Schädelbasis. Virchows Archiv 298:195–227
27. Nadol JB (1977) Electron microscopicobservation in a case of long-standing profound sensorineural deafness. Ann Otol Rhinol Laryngol 86:507–517
28. Fraysse BG (1980) Ménière's disease and endolymphatic hydrops. Ann Otol Rhinol Laryngol 89 [Suppl 76] 1–22
29. De Moura L (1969) Further observations on acoustic neurinoma. Trans Pa Acad Ophthalmol Otolaryngol 73:60
30. Gussan R, Adkins JW (1974) Saccule degeneration and ductus runiens obstruction. Arch Otolaryngol 99:132–135
31. Sakata F (1963) Pathophysiology of Ménière's disease (in Japanese). J Otolaryngol Jpn 35:609–618
32. Rizvi SS, Gibbin KP (1979) Effect of transverse temporal bone fracture on the fluid compartment of the inner ear. Ann Otol Rhinol Laryngol 88:741–748
33. Schuknecht HF (1973) Pathology in a case of profound congenital deafness. J Laryngol Otol 87:947–955
34. Schuknecht HF (1980) Mondini dysplasia. Ann Otol Rhinol Laryngol 89 [Suppl 65]: 1–23
35. Lindsay JR, Hinojosa R (1978) Ear anomalies associated with renal dysplasia and immunodeficiency disease. Ann Otol Rhinol Laryngol 87:10–17
36. Gussen R (1980) Endolymphatic hydrops with absence of vein in paravestibular canaliculus. Ann Otol Rhinol Laryngol 89:157–161
37. Gussen RS (1968) Mondini type of genetically determined deafness. J Laryngol Otol 82:41–55

Subject Index